Fibroblasts - Advances in Inflammation, Autoimmunity and Cancer

Edited by Mojca Frank Bertoncelj and Katja Lakota

Published in London, United Kingdom

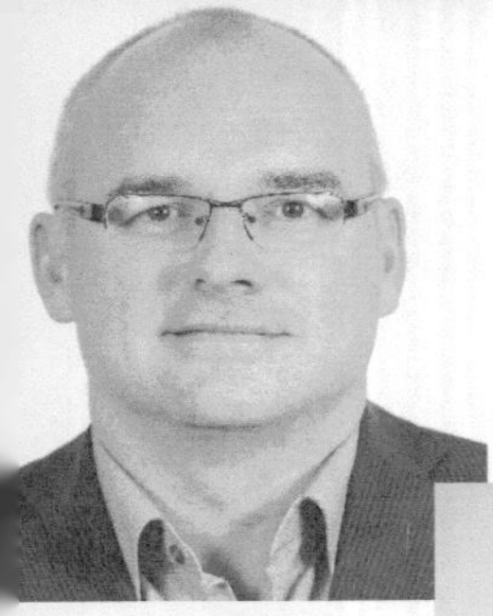
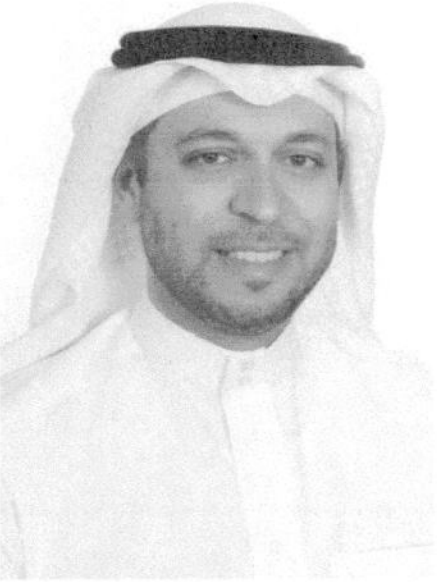
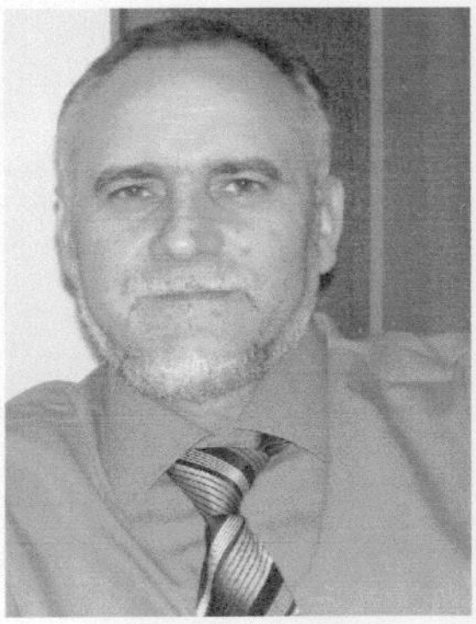
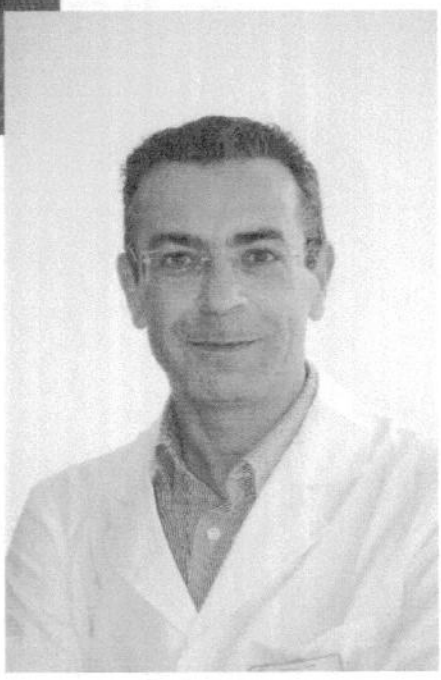
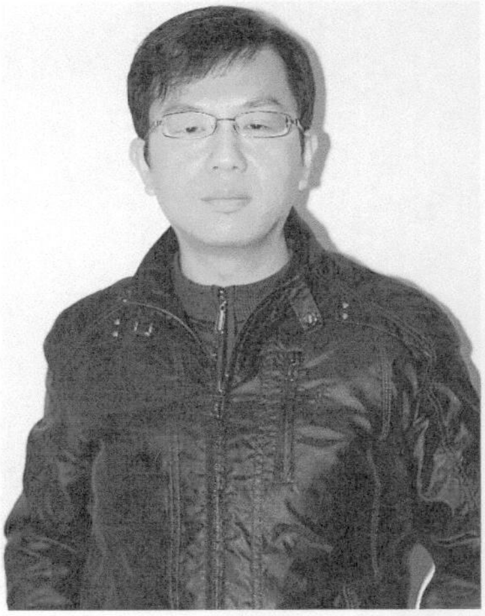
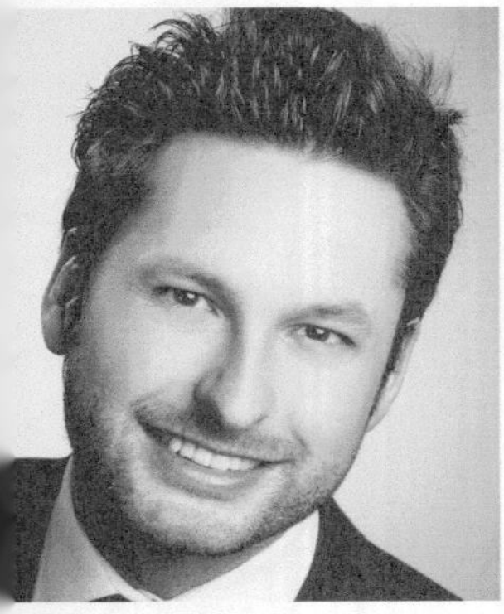
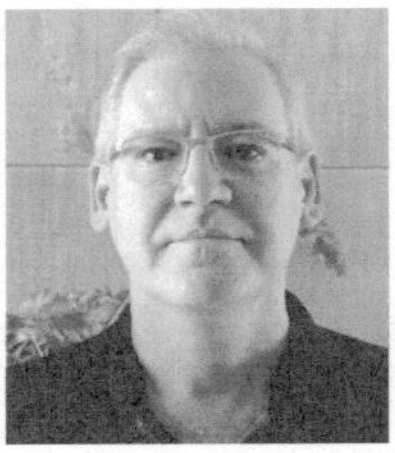

IntechOpen

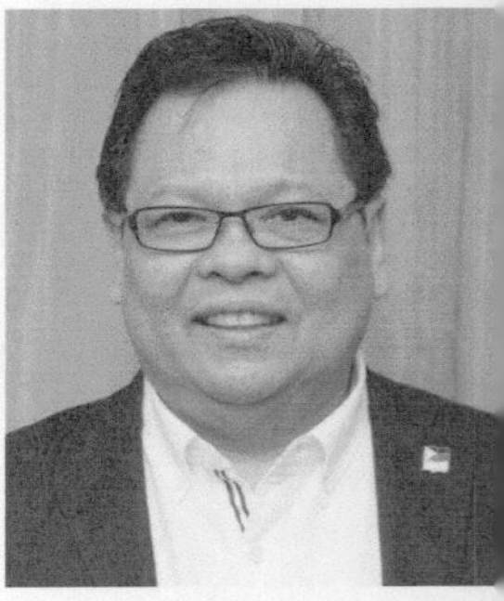
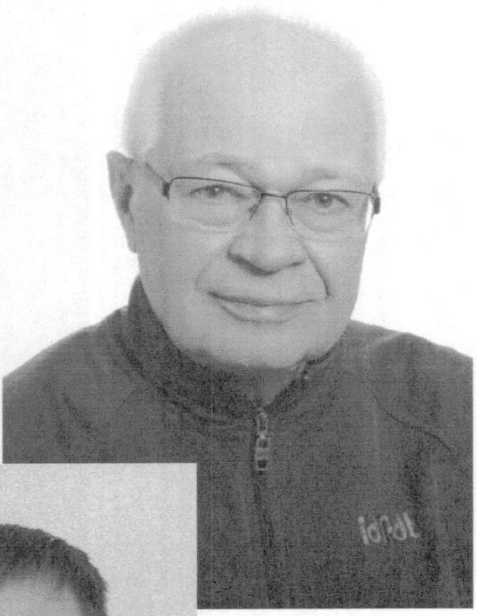
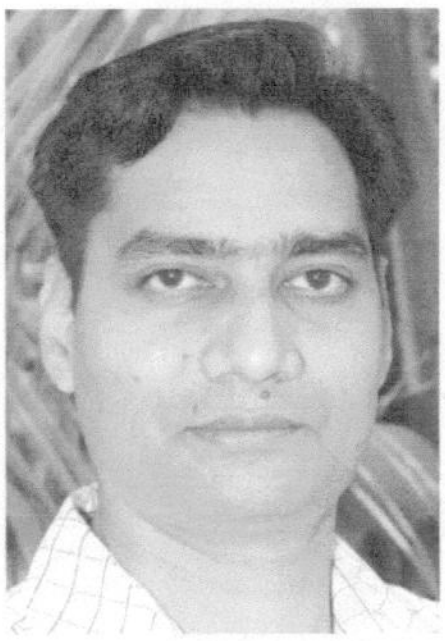
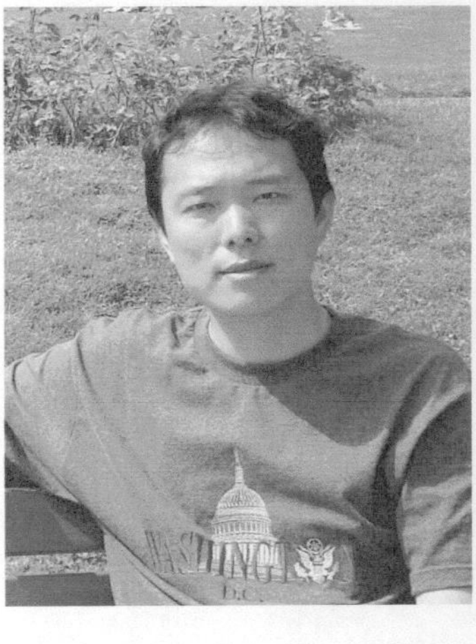
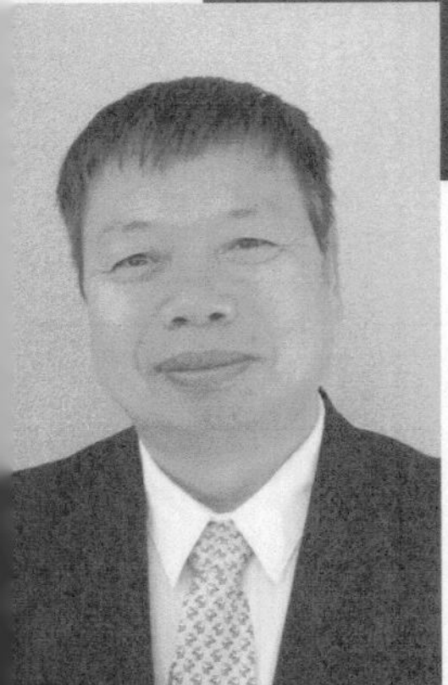
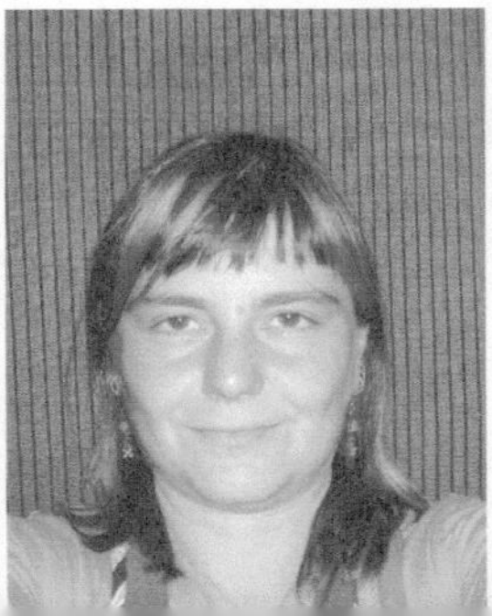

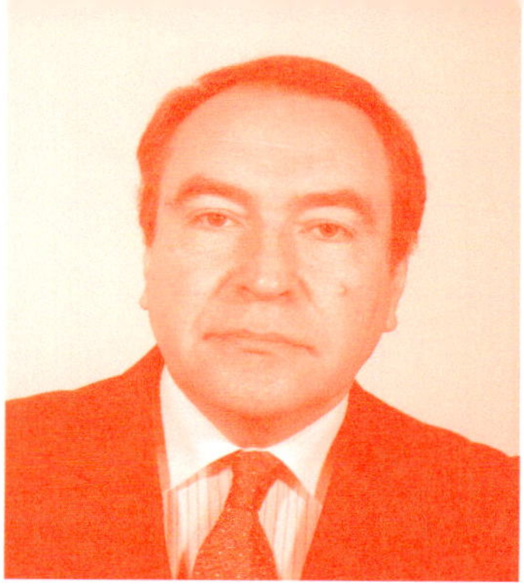
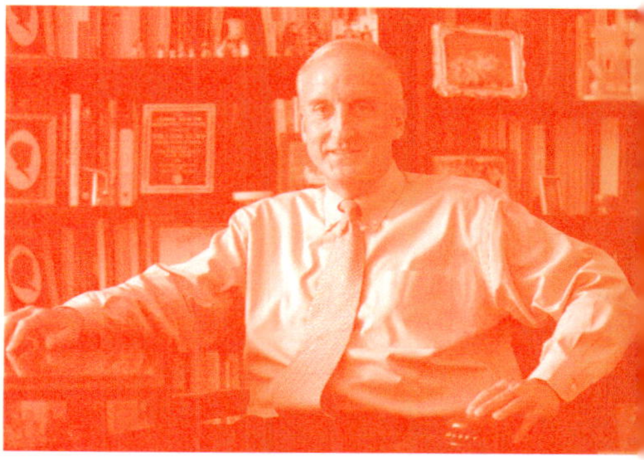
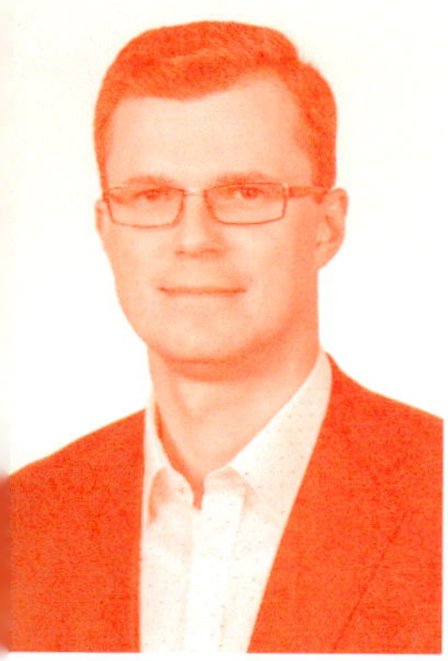
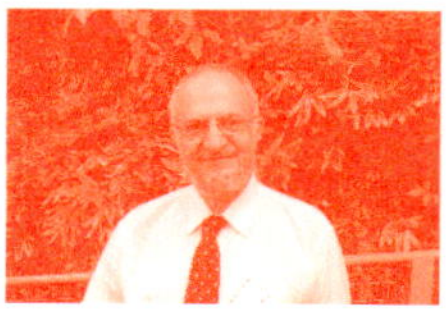
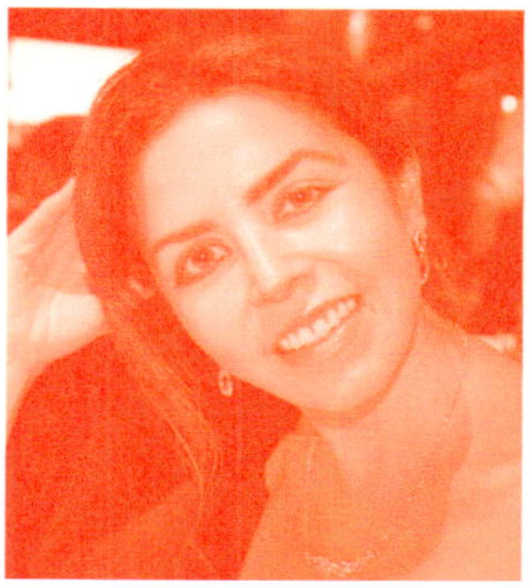

Supporting open minds since 2005

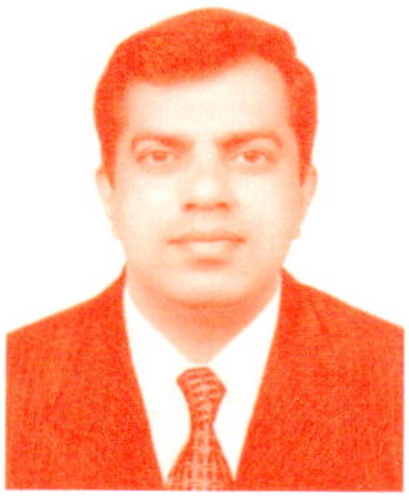
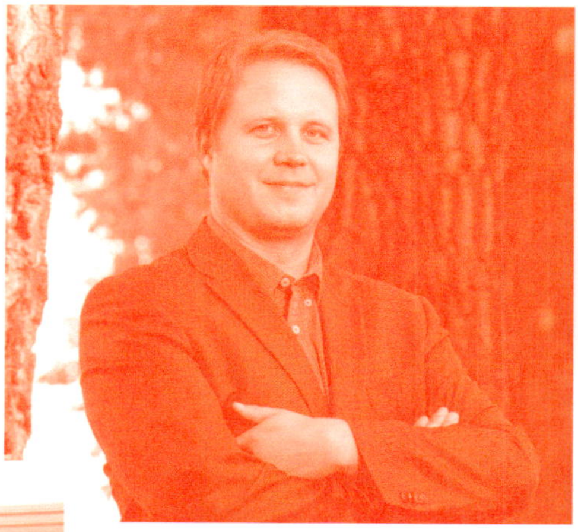
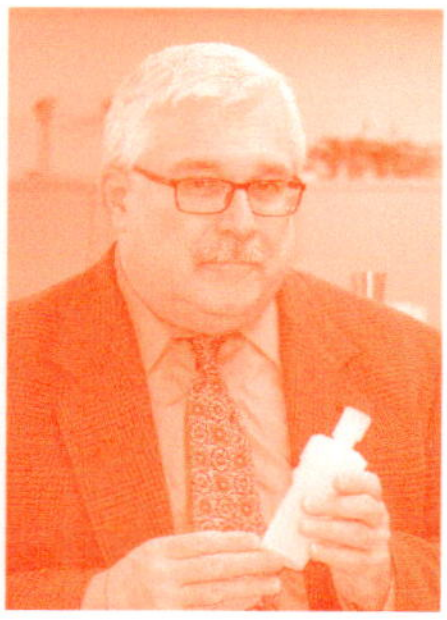
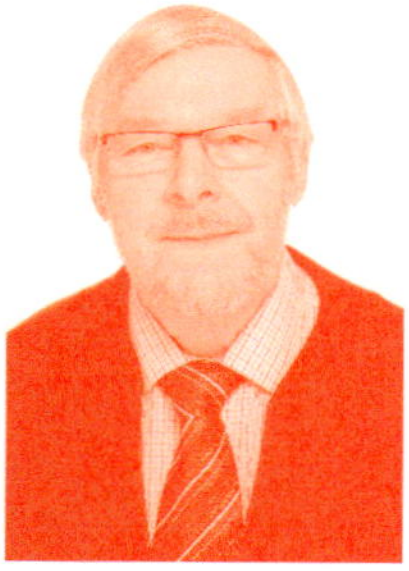
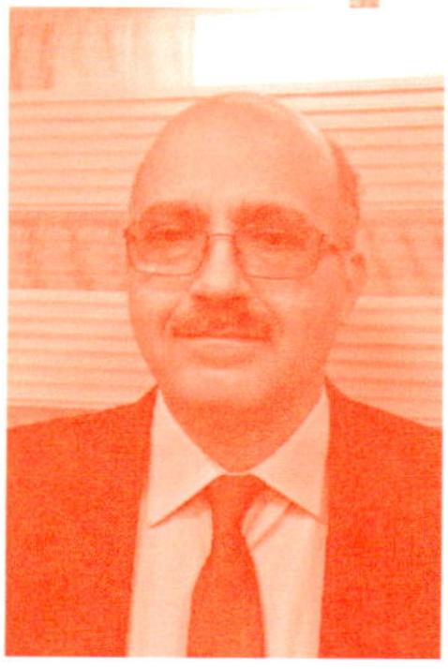
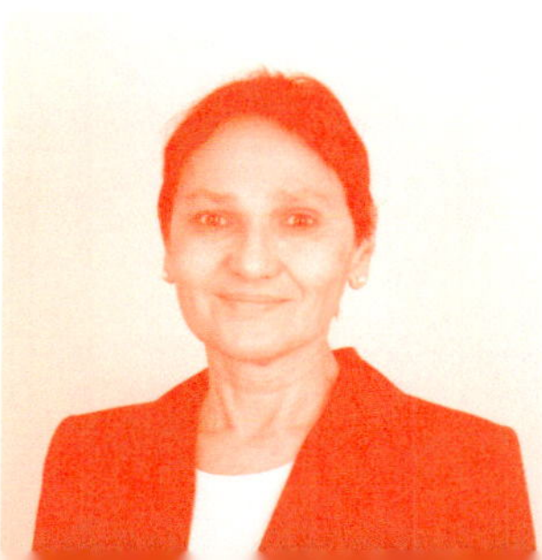
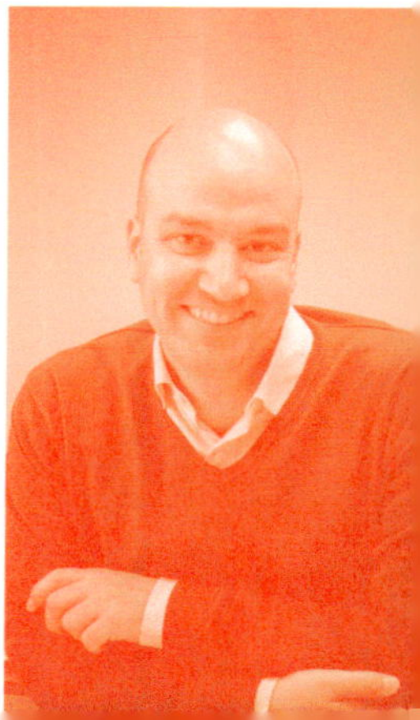

Fibroblasts - Advances in Inflammation, Autoimmunity and Cancer
http://dx.doi.org/10.5772/intechopen.87462
Edited by Mojca Frank Bertoncelj and Katja Lakota

Part of IntechOpen Book Series: Biochemistry, Volume 25
Book Series Editor: Miroslav Blumenberg

Contributors
Tue Kragstrup, Søren Lomholt, Morten Aagaard Nielsen, Maithri Aspari, Peter Bjørnlund Jørgensen, Christopher Buckley, Adam Croft, Tadeja Kuret, Snežna Sodin-Šemrl, Kerstin Klein, Janja Zupan, Caroline Ospelt, Masoumeh Mirrahimi, Motoko Yanagita, Takahisa Yoshikawa, Yuki Sato

First published in London, United Kingdom, 2021 by IntechOpen
IntechOpen is the global imprint of INTECHOPEN LIMITED, registered in England and Wales, registration number: 11086078, 5 Princes Gate Court, London, SW7 2QJ, United Kingdom
Printed in Croatia

British Library Cataloguing-in-Publication Data
A catalogue record for this book is available from the British Library

Additional hard and PDF copies can be obtained from orders@intechopen.com

Fibroblasts - Advances in Inflammation, Autoimmunity and Cancer
Edited by Mojca Frank Bertoncelj and Katja Lakota
p. cm.
Print ISBN 978-1-78985-799-3
Online ISBN 978-1-78985-800-6
eBook (PDF) ISBN 978-1-83880-578-4
ISSN 2632-0983

For EU product safety concerns:
IN TECH d.o.o., Prolaz Marije Krucifikse Kozulić 3, 51000 Rijeka, Croatia, info@intechopen.com or visit our website at intechopen.com.

IntechOpen Book Series
Biochemistry
Volume 25

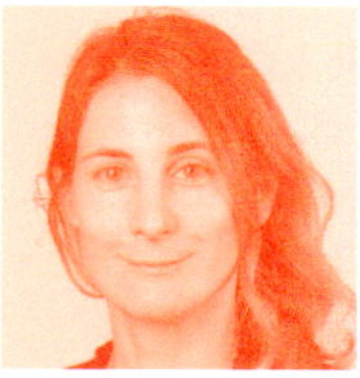

Mojca Frank Bertoncelj, MD, Ph.D., is a group leader of the research team "Protective Tissue Factors in Autoimmune Diseases" at BioMed X Institute, Heidelberg, Germany, developing 3-D models of human synovium and exploring molecular mechanisms of resolution of inflammation in chronic inflammatory diseases. She holds a doctorate in Biomedicine at the University of Ljubljana, Slovenia, serves as a guest lecturer at the University of Primorska, Slovenia and is a VTIS society mentor for young talents in life sciences. She is a winner of BioMed X's innovation boot camp and a recipient of the Walter-Siegenthaler Medaille in Silber for arthritis research. Before joining BioMed X, she was a junior group leader of the Integrative biology of immune-mediated inflammatory diseases team at the University Hospital Zurich/the University of Zurich, Switzerland.

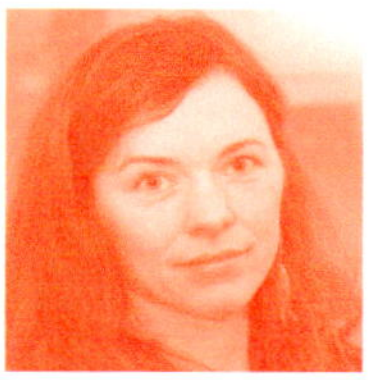

Assistant Professor Katja Lakota, MPharm, Ph.D., received her doctorate in Biomedicine in 2014 at the Faculty of Pharmacy, University of Ljubljana. She is a senior scientist at the Department of Rheumatology, University Medical Centre Ljubljana, Slovenia. As a Fulbright scholar, she spent a research year in the laboratory of Professor John Varga at the Northwestern University, Chicago, studying the role of adiponectin anti-fibrotic signalling in fibroblasts. She investigated mechanisms leading to fibrosis development in systemic sclerosis in a postdoctoral fellowship awarded in 2018 by Slovenian Research Agency. Dr. Lakota is an assistant professor at the University of Primorska, Faculty of Mathematics, Natural Sciences and Information Technologies, Slovenia, holding courses on structures of biological molecules and systems biology in human diseases in the undergraduate study program bioinformatics.

Editors of Volume 25:
Mojca Frank Bertoncelj
BioMed X Institute, Heidelberg, Germany

Katja Lakota
Department of Rheumatology, University Medical Centre (UCM) Ljubljana, Ljubljana, Slovenia

Book Series Editor: Miroslav Blumenberg
NYU Langone Medical Center, New York, USA

Scope of the Series

Biochemistry, the study of chemical transformations occurring within living organisms, impacts all of the life sciences, from molecular crystallography and genetics, to ecology, medicine and population biology. Biochemistry studies macromolecules - proteins, nucleic acids, carbohydrates and lipids –their building blocks, structures, functions and interactions. Much of biochemistry is devoted to enzymes, proteins that catalyze chemical reactions, enzyme structures, mechanisms of action and their roles within cells. Biochemistry also studies small signaling molecules, coenzymes, inhibitors, vitamins and hormones, which play roles in the life process. Biochemical experimentation, besides coopting the methods of classical chemistry, e.g., chromatography, adopted new techniques, e.g., X-ray diffraction, electron microscopy, NMR, radioisotopes, and developed sophisticated microbial genetic tools, e.g., auxotroph mutants and their revertants, fermentation, etc. More recently, biochemistry embraced the 'big data' omics systems.

Initial biochemical studies have been exclusively analytic: dissecting, purifying and examining individual components of a biological system; in exemplary words of Efraim Racker, (1913 –1991) "Don't waste clean thinking on dirty enzymes." Today, however, biochemistry is becoming more agglomerative and comprehensive, setting out to integrate and describe fully a particular biological system. The 'big data' metabolomics can define the complement of small molecules, e.g., in a soil or biofilm sample; proteomics can distinguish all the proteins comprising e.g., serum; metagenomics can identify all the genes in a complex environment e.g., the bovine rumen. This Biochemistry Series will address both the current research on biomolecules, and the emerging trends with great promise.

Contents

Preface XI

Section 1
General Principles of Fibroblast and Mesenchymal Stem Cell Biology in Health and Disease 1

Chapter 1 3
Organ- and Site-Specific HOX Gene Expression in Stromal Cells
by Masoumeh Mirrahimi and Caroline Ospelt

Chapter 2 21
Mesenchymal Stem/Stromal Cells and Fibroblasts: Their Roles in Tissue Injury and Regeneration, and Age-Related Degeneration
by Janja Zupan

Section 2
Unique and Shared Fibroblast Mechanisms across Human Tissues and Pathologies 47

Chapter 3 49
The Role of Fibroblasts in Atherosclerosis Progression
by Tadeja Kuret and Snežna Sodin-Šemrl

Chapter 4 69
Heterogeneity of Fibroblasts in Healthy and Diseased Kidneys
by Takahisa Yoshikawa, Yuki Sato and Motoko Yanagita

Chapter 5 85
Fibroblast-Like Synovial Cell Subsets in Rheumatoid Arthritis
by Søren Lomholt, Morten A. Nielsen, Maithri P. Aspari, Peter B. Jørgensen, Adam P. Croft, Christopher Buckley and Tue W. Kragstrup

Chapter 6 105
Fibroblasts in Sjögren's Syndrome
by Kerstin Klein

Preface

Fibroblasts are vital structural cells of the human body with core roles in tissue homeostasis and disease. While primarily recognised as producers of extracellular matrix and central effectors in wound healing, using them as a feeder layer in cell culturing sheds some understanding on their nurturing roles for other cell types. Recent years have brought remarkable advances in molecular and functional characterisation of fibroblasts, decoding their organ and sub-tissular niche specificity, anatomical sub-specialisation, reactivity, heterogeneity and plasticity across the human body in health and disease. This knowledge substantially changed our conventional view about fibroblast roles in human disease. In 2021, fibroblasts are being widely recognised for their active contribution to chronicity, recurrence, progression and therapeutic resistance against many human pathologies, including chronic inflammatory and systemic autoimmune diseases and cancer.

This book provides essential insights into shared and unique characteristics of fibroblasts and mesenchymal stem cells across the body and their crosstalk with the innate and adaptive immune systems, other tissue-resident cells and cancer cells. The book explains the roles of fibroblasts and mesenchymal stem cells in shaping tissue microenvironments and structural immunity and discusses the recent discoveries about their pathogenic actions in tissue remodelling, repair, inflammation, angiogenesis or lymphangiogenesis, particularly in autoimmune diseases and cancer. The first two chapters uncover the general principles of fibroblast and mesenchymal stem cell biology and pathobiology, followed by a focused insight into shared and unique characteristics of exocrine, vascular, synovial and salivary gland fibroblasts in the following four chapters.

Chapter 1, *Organ- and Site-Specific HOX Gene Expression in Stromal Cells*, delves into the embryonically imprinted positional memory of tissue-resident fibroblasts with a principal focus on the coding and non-coding genes in the HOX clusters. Professor Ospelt and colleagues discuss the contribution of epigenetic mechanisms to the location-specific fibroblast imprinting across the human body and furthermore, review the implication of site-specific fibroblast memories for organ-specific tropism of human pathologies, such as arthritis and cancer—the seed and soil principle. In Chapter 2, *Mesenchymal Stem/Stromal Cells and Fibroblasts: Their Roles in Tissue Injury and Regeneration, and Age-Related Degeneration*, Assistant Professor Zupan introduces and aligns the characteristics of tissue-resident fibroblasts and tissue-derived mesenchymal stem cells in homeostatic and pathological conditions, including injury and age-related tissue degeneration. Both cell types crucially control and contribute to the regeneration of skin, ligaments, joints, bone and other tissues and have potent immunomodulatory roles, enabling a successful cessation of the inflammatory process. Boosting the complementary roles of mesenchymal stem cells and fibroblasts could be therapeutically exploited for tissue regeneration. Chapter 3, *The Role of Fibroblasts in Atherosclerosis Progression*, offers further insights into the associations between stem cells and fibroblasts from a perspective of an arterial wall. Professor Šemrl and colleagues discuss a challenging delineation between stem cells and fibroblasts at the adventitia/media niche and summarise the heterogeneity of vessel wall fibroblasts. Adventitial fibroblasts, populating healthy vessel walls, characteristically migrate to and invade the media and intima of the injured or stress vessels. These cells then drive neointima formation, can transdifferentiate into extracellular matrix-depositing myofibroblasts, promote adventitial neovascularisation and regulate immune cell infiltration, thus crucially contributing to vascular pathologies, such as atherosclerosis and pulmonary artery hypertension. In Chapter 4, *Heterogeneity of Fibroblasts in Healthy and Diseased Kidneys*, the book's focus steers from the vascular towards kidney fibroblasts and their pronounced regional and functional heterogeneity. A small subset of corticomedullary fibroblasts that express erythropoietin and control erythropoiesis exemplifies this regional specialisation of kidney fibroblasts. Professor Yanagita and colleagues re-examine the dual roles of kidney fibroblasts, particularly their contribution to renal tubule regeneration contrasted by their pathogenic roles in kidney fibrosis and inflammation, and discuss fibroblast roles in the formation of the tertiary lymphoid structures in chronic kidney diseases and rheumatoid arthritis, and Sjögren's syndrome as part of the succeeding chapter. In Chapter 5, *Fibroblast-Like Synovial Cell Subsets in Rheumatoid Arthritis*, Associate Professor Kragstrup and colleagues present the recent discoveries about the diversity of fibroblast-like synoviocytes/synovial fibroblasts in rheumatoid arthritis based on single-cell RNA-sequencing studies. Synovial fibroblast functions in the initiation and persistence of synovial inflammation and joint destruction are illuminated. The authors review the evidence about the roles of lining CD55+ synovial fibroblasts in cartilage and bone destruction, depict the enrichment of the proinflammatory sublining THY1+ synovial fibroblasts in rheumatoid arthritis and propose potential fibroblast markers for the development of targeted treatments. Moving from the autoimmune diseases of the synovial joints to the autoimmune diseases of the exocrine glands, Chapter 6, *Fibroblasts in Sjögren's Syndrome*, emphasises the inflammatory, immunomodulatory and regenerative functions of salivary gland fibroblasts in Sjögren's syndrome, a chronic inflammatory autoimmune disease of the exocrine glands. The chapter describes specific fibroblast subsets that drive the formation of tertiary lymphoid structures associated with disease severity and risk of lymphoma development. Dr. Klein wraps up the chapter with the recently introduced concept of an inflammatory fibroblast phenotype shared across many chronic immune-mediated inflammatory diseases. This concept excellently repercusses the overall book's goal of utilising expanding fibroblast knowledge to develop the pathology-based patient classification and propose novel therapies beyond disease boundaries.

Mojca Frank Bertoncelj
BioMed X Institute,
Heidelberg, Germany

Katja Lakota
Department of Rheumatology,
University Medical Centre (UCM) Ljubljana,
Ljubljana, Slovenia

Section 1

General Principles of Fibroblast and Mesenchymal Stem Cell Biology in Health and Disease

Chapter 1

Organ- and Site-Specific HOX Gene Expression in Stromal Cells

Masoumeh Mirrahimi and Caroline Ospelt

Abstract

HOX genes are a group of evolutionarily conserved genes that encode a family of transcription factors that regulate early developmental morphogenetic processes and continue to be expressed into adulthood. These highly conserved HOX factors play an unquestioned crucial role as master regulators during embryonic vertebrate development and morphogenesis by controlling the three dimensional body plan organization. HOX genes specify regions of the body plan of an embryo along the head-tail axis. They encode proteins that specify the characteristics of 'position', ensuring that the correct structures form in the correct places of the body. Expression of HOX is known to persist in many tissues in the postnatal period suggesting the role of these genes not only during development but also for the functioning of tissues throughout life. The tissue-specific pattern of HOX gene expression is inherent in stromal/stem cells of mesenchymal origin, such as mesenchymal stromal cells, fibroblasts, smooth muscle cells, and preadipocytes, enabling them to memorize their topographic location in the form of their HOX code and to fulfill their location-specific functions. In this chapter, we focus on the expression and potential role of HOX genes in adult tissues. We review evidence that site-specific expression of HOX genes is connected to location-specific disease susceptibility and review studies showing that dysregulated expression of HOX genes can be associated with various diseases. By recognizing the importance of site-specific molecular mechanisms in the organ stroma, we gain new insights into the processes underlying the site-specific manifestation of disease.

Keywords: Fibroblasts, HOX genes, site-specific gene expression, embryonic development, disease locations

1. Introduction

In vertebrate animals, the stromal compartment of organs is composed of extracellular matrix and mesenchymal cells. Fibroblasts are one of the most abundant and principal stromal cell types and have a variety of vital, locally specialized functions in tissue repair and homeostasis. Primarily, they are the main source of extracellular matrix (ECM) proteins, which, in addition to providing a structural scaffold for cells, play critical roles in determining cell phenotype and function. Fibroblasts produce and secrete all components of the ECM, including structural proteins, adhesive proteins, and a space-filling ground substance composed of glycosaminoglycans and proteoglycans [1].

Furthermore, as a result of their reciprocal interaction with epithelial cells, fibroblast cells play an important role during development and morphogenesis of tissues and organs including the skin, eyes, lung and other visceral organs. The organ stroma provides a structural framework and guidance for blood and lymphatic vessels, nerves and leukocytes and is critically involved in the regulation of physiological organ function.

During stress, fibroblasts respond by sending signals to help the surrounding tissue to adapt to changes in the environment [2]. The phenotype of fibroblast can transform and provides the necessary components to replace wounded tissue. During pathologic states, however, ECM can be generated in excessive quantities, leading to irreversible organ dysfunction caused by collagen deposition in a dysregulated manner [3].

Given the wide variations of gene expression and strikingly different responses to extracellular signals among fibroblasts from different organs, these fibroblast populations should be considered as distinct cell types. Human fibroblasts obtained from vocal fold, trachea, lung, abdomen, scalp, upper gingiva, and soft palate, displayed a phenomenon of global topographic differentiation across all anatomic site domains with the specialized genotype of the vocal fold fibroblast uniquely characterized to achieve homeostasis under complex mechanobiological requirements [4].

During development of multicellular organisms, developmental control genes are critical for pattern formation and cell fate specification in specific spatiotemporal patterns [5]. Most of these genes encode transcription factors acting in cascades and networks, regulating the expression of further developmental control genes and ultimately organ-specific 'effector' genes, which control patterning, morphogenesis and differentiation of tissue-specific functions and specific body parts [6]. The wide range of organ specific differences in fibroblast function is complemented by distinct and characteristic gene expression patterns depending on their anatomic site of origin [7]. Examples include HOX genes, which can lead to the transformation of specific body segments when mutated [8], Pax6, which controls eye development [9] and MyoD, which is crucial for muscle formation [10].

Functional diversity of fibroblasts is not only important during embryonic developmental and physiologic specialization of many tissues, but might also influence site- and organ-specific differences in the susceptibility of different tissues to disease development [11, 12].

2. Site-specific regulation of gene expression by HOX genes

Spatial organization of cellular differentiation is achieved by a unique local developmental specification of cell types. This can be reinforced by the cells' interpretation of environmental signals specific to their position in the body. HOX genes are known to be master regulators of body pattern formation during embryogenesis, activating other genes to specify positional identities in development.

In humans, there are 39 HOX genes organized into 4 distinct clusters. The 4 clusters map to 4 different chromosomes and contain between 9 and 11 genes. These clusters, labeled HOXA, HOXB, HOXC and HOXD, are located on chromosomes 7p14, 17q21, 12q13 and 2q31, respectively [13, 14]. HOX proteins are transcription factors that are bound by different protein cofactors. The analysis of HOX protein binding activity showed that the homeodomain, a highly conserved 60 amino acid helix-turn-helix motif, is a DNA-binding protein that recognize AT rich short DNA motifs, often with a core of TAAT [15]. In several cases, functional specificity of the different HOX proteins could be attributed to the homeodomain itself [16, 17]. The homeodomains showed distinct protein- and/or DNA-binding activities, suggesting that variation in sequence recognition may be a factor in their functional diversity.

In vertebrates, the different sets of HOX genes are expressed in parallel [15]. Thus, site- and/or organ-specific fibroblast phenotypes are shaped by a combinatorial expression of genes from the four HOX clusters. Genome-wide gene expression profile of 47 fibroblast populations from 43 anatomic sites spanning the human body, including arm, leg, trunk, foreskin and internal organs, analyzed by unsupervised hierarchical clustering revealed a specific code of HOX genes according to their position in the human body. Fibroblasts from the same topographic site, independent from which organ they were isolated, expressed the same, site-specific, unique "HOX-code", which resulted in grouping of the cells from the same site together, based solely on the expression pattern of the HOX genes. This suggests that the expression of a specific set of HOX genes is connected to the cells' location in the body, potentially conferring important site-specific functions needed in a particular location [18].

Thus, site-specific variations in the gene expression programs of fibroblasts are not random but are systematically related to their positional identities along the major anatomical axes, which are formed during embryogenesis.

3. The role of HOX genes in embryonic development

In many animals, especially vertebrates, various HOX gene paralogues are located genetically close to each other in clusters [19]. The order of the genes on the chromosome corresponds to the expression of the genes in the developing embryo [14, 20, 21]. Thereby, the genes in the 5′ genetic locus are expressed in the anterior end or distal parts of the developing organism and the genes in the 3′ locus are expressed in the posterior end or proximal parts - a phenomenon known as spatial colinearity [22]. In addition, there is a temporal sequence of activation of HOX genes in vertebrate. 5′ genes are expressed later, whereas 3′ genes are expressed earlier in embryonic development [18, 19]. The unique orderly arrangement of the genes in the genome is related to the activation of HOX genes in a temporal sequence by gradual unpacking of chromatin along a gene cluster, thereby controlling the expression of the right HOX gene at the right location at the right time in embryogenesis [23]. The temporal and spatial tightly controlled expression of HOX genes in mesenchymal cells can thus explain how genetic information is translated to the spatial organization of various cells in the body (**Figure 1**).

Over the past years, gain-of-function and loss-of-function approaches in chick and mice together with studies of mutations, indicated the essential role of HOX genes in proper vertebrate limb growth and organization of the structures within both the anterior-to-posterior axis and the proximal-to-distal axis. The resultant phenotypes typically follow the expected spatio-temporal expression of HOX genes with more 3′ genes causing malformations in more anterior and proximal areas and more 5′ genes causing defects in more posterior, distal body segments and organs. For instance, Hoxa13 and Hoxd13 have been identified to be involved in endochondral bone formation [24]. HOXD13 is mutated in synpolydactyly, and HOXA13 is mutated in Hand-Foot-Genital syndrome [22]. Overexpression of Hoxa13 affects the expression of Enpp2, an enzyme produced in precartilaginous condensations that modulates cell motility [25]. Loss-of-function of Hoxa13 was also reported to modulate expression of bone morphogenetic proteins like BMP2 and BMP7 [26]. Hoxa13 regulated expression of BMP2 and BMP7 was shown to control distal limb morphogenesis [27].

Temporal and spatial dynamic regulation of gene expression is a hallmark of developmental control genes, since they have to act locally in order to affect specific developmental processes [28]. By linking differentiation programs to specific cell

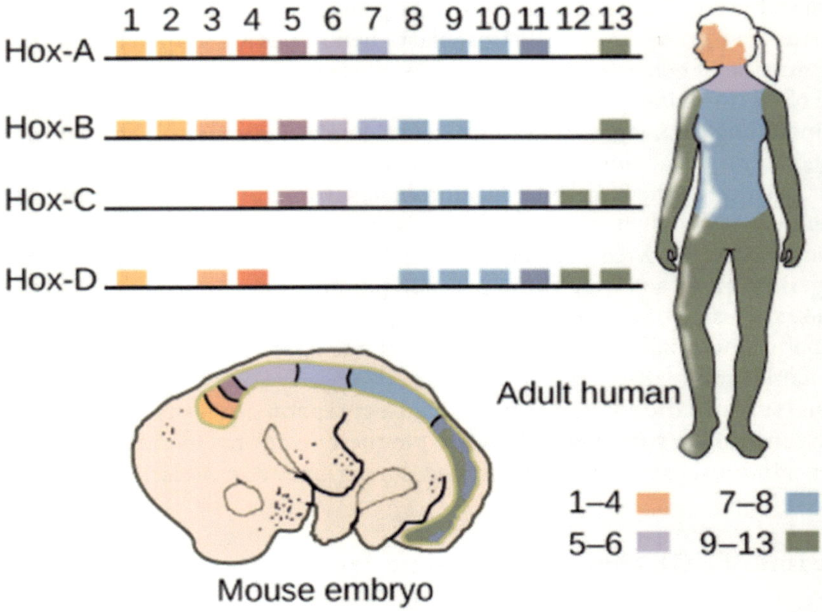

Figure 1.
The spatial organization of the Hox genes in the various genomic Hox clusters (Hox-A, Hox-B, Hox-C and Hox-D) is tightly linked to the pattern of their expression in the embryo (mouse embryo shown here). The same pattern of HOX gene expression that formed during embryonic development can still be found in stromal tissues (fibroblasts, endothelial cells) in the adult human body. The picture was taken from the course 'Homeotic genes' by the Khan Academy. Note: All Khan Academy content is available for free at www.khanacademy.org.

positions, selected cells can be programmed to develop similarly in a defined region. While spatial boundaries are first defined during embryonic development, these spatial patterns of cellular specialization also need to be maintained throughout adulthood as the tissues undergo continuous self-renewal.

4. Epigenetic regulation of HOX gene expression

Epigenetic mechanisms have an important role in the regulation of HOX gene expression in embryonic development and in differentiated cells. The established expression patterns of HOX genes must be precisely and clonally maintained throughout development. Epigenetic regulation of gene expression by chromatin structure is defined by a set of posttranslational modifications of histones, such as methylation, acetylation and phosphorylation. Furthermore, gene expression can be epigenetically regulated by DNA methylation.

In totipotent embryonic stem cells, HOX genes are silenced and then rapidly activated during embryogenesis. In drosophila and vertebrates, repressive Polycomb and Trithorax group complexes regulating histone methylation control the proper maintenance of HOX gene expression during this process [29]. Tight temporal and spatial control of HOX gene expression in this phase is essential. In vertebrates, dynamic changes in histone methylation are observed during the sequential activation of HOX genes in the embryo, suggesting that progressive change of epigenetic modifications regulate collinear gene activation in these loci [29]. Based on the presence of retinoic acid response elements (RAREs) in the regulatory region of many of the HOX genes, it was shown that that retinoic acid is a crucial factor in the epigenetic regulation of histone methylation of the clustered HOX genes [30].

During developmental stages, the genetic loci of the 4 HOX clusters carry so-called "bivalent chromatin tags", like many other key developmental genes in embryonic stem cells [31]. This means that the HOX clusters possess at the same time "active" (i.e., trimethylation of histone 3 at lysine 4 -H3K4me3) and "inactive" (i.e., trimethylation of histone 3 at lysine 27 -H3K27me3) histone marks. In the presence of the right trans-acting factors, these bivalent tags can rapidly change to allow binding to cis-elements and initiation of transcription [32].

Epigenetic modifications also regulate tissue specific expression of HOX genes and mesenchymal cell differentiation [33]. In a study of genome-wide differential DNA methylation by reduced representation bisulfite sequencing (RRBS), the HOX gene clusters were highly overrepresented among the genes with hypermethylation in the skeletal muscle lineage [34]. Analysis of DNA methylation of HOX genes in myoblasts, myotubes and adult skeletal muscle tissue revealed that myogenic DNA hypermethylation of promoters and enhancers of HOX genes helps to fine-tune HOX gene expression in cellular differentiation [34].

HOX loci contain many noncoding transcripts. Long non-coding RNAs (lncRNAs) represent a class of noncoding RNAs that are longer than 200 nucleotides without protein-coding potential. They have been found to function as master regulators of gene expression in health and in various human diseases. LncRNAs can regulate biological functions in cis and in trans [35]. For instance, they can recruit histone modifying enzymes to specific genomic sites and serve as scaffolds for gene expression modulating enzymes [36].

HOX antisense intergenic RNA (HOTAIR) is a lncRNA that is encoded in the HOXC locus and that mediates the placement of repressive H3K27me3 marks. HOTAIR expression has been shown to repress the expression of genes in the 3' HOXD locus and thus was suggested to be an important epigenetic regulator of site-specific HOX expression during embryonic development [37]. However, these data is debated and the full role of HOTAIR in embryonic development is not yet understood [38].

HOXA transcript at the distal tip (HOTTIP) is a 3764 nucleotide lncRNA encoded from a genomic region in the 5′ tip of the HOXA locus, regulating the expression of HOXA13 [39]. By binding the adaptor protein WD repeat-containing protein 5 (WDR5) and interaction with mixed lineage leukemia (MLL), HOTTIP can catalyze methylation of histone H3 lysine K4 (H3K4). H3K4 methylation is associated with increased gene transcription and MLL-WDR5 complexes were shown to occupy transcriptional start sites of various HOXA genes.

To date, the complex epigenetic patterns of cellular specialization in adult vertebrates and the mechanisms of their maintenance are not well understood. Epigenetic conservation of region-specific HOX gene expression in human adult fibroblasts suggests that they serve to maintain the differential patterns of the stroma during homeostasis and regeneration [40].

5. HOX gene expression in specific fibroblast populations

5.1 Skin fibroblasts

Epithelial tissues such as skin demonstrate remarkable anatomic differences leading to diversity on their structure and function. Genome-wide studies in skin fibroblasts demonstrated that site-specific HOX expression in these cells can define and maintain skin positional identity [41]. Analysis of genome-wide patterns of gene expression in cultured fetal and adult human skin fibroblasts at different anatomical sites showed distinct and characteristic site-specific transcriptional patterns, suggesting that fibroblasts at different locations in the body possess specialized functions [7]. The maintenance of region-specific HOX gene expression in adult fibroblasts may serve as a source of positional memory for skin during homeostasis and regeneration.

For instance, HOXA13, a gene that is preferentially expressed at distal body parts such as hands and feet, remains essential for maintaining the distal-specific transcriptional program in adult fibroblasts by inducing the expression of WNT5A, which is crucial for distal organ development [41]. Furthermore, reduction of HOXA13 abrogates the ability of distal fibroblasts to produce epidermal keratin 9, a distal-specific gene. Keratin 9 has been shown to be important for maintaining the mechanical integrity of palmar and plantar skin [42]. Together these observations suggest that HOXA13-regulated gene expression in adult human fibroblasts provide the specific functions of plantar and palmar skin.

5.2 Synovial fibroblasts

Synovial fibroblasts are crucially involved in inflammation and joint destruction in chronic joint inflammation (arthritis) [43]. Synovial fibroblasts isolated from different joint locations show substantial differences in their transcriptome and function, in particular a site-specific HOX gene signature was found [44]. Adult human and mouse SFs from different anatomical locations exhibit joint-specific HOXA and HOXC signatures that are maintained over several passages in cell culture conditions, are arthritis independent and reproduced in whole synovial tissues.

This HOX gene signature was shown to be epigenetically imprinted by DNA methylation and histone modifications [44, 45]. The joint-specific HOX expression in mouse and human synovial fibroblasts and synovial tissues reflected the pattern of HOX gene expression during embryonic limb development [44]. Only few studies explored the functional role of different HOX proteins in synovial fibroblasts. HOXD10 silencing downregulated the p38/c-Jun N-terminal kinase signaling pathway, and suppressed the migration of synovial fibroblasts [26]. HOXD9 was found to modulate proliferation of synovial fibroblasts [46]. During development of the distal limb mesenchyme, Hoxd13 is the most strongly expressed HoxD gene, with a progressive decline in expression levels of Hoxd12 to Hoxd9 [47]. Moreover, in tetrapods, coordinated expression of the 5′ located Hoxd genes is essential for the development of digits [48]. Thus, site-specific expression of HOXD genes in distal joints (hands and feet) [44] might influence the activation of pro-inflammatory pathways and the migratory and proliferative capacity of synovial fibroblasts. Notably, distal joints are the first and most severely affected joints in patients with rheumatoid arthritis (RA).

Other HOX genes may also play a critical role in the pathogenesis of RA. One study showed that basic fibroblast growth factor (bFGF) affects the expression and transcriptional regulation of HOXC4 and via this pathway promotes hyperplasia of the synovium in RA [49].

Several studies suggest epigenetic changes as determinants of a persistent activated phenotype of synovial fibroblasts in RA [43]. RA synovial fibroblasts display wide-spread changes in DNA methylation causing up-regulation of disease relevant genes such as growth factors, adhesion molecules and matrix-metalloproteinases (MMPs) [50–52]. The tight epigenetic regulation of site-specific HOX gene expression might thus be disturbed in RA synovial fibroblasts, leading to aberrant expression of HOX genes at sites where they are normally repressed. The expression of HOXD10 for instance was found to be higher in knee synovial fibroblasts from patients with rheumatoid arthritis (RA) compared to osteoarthritis (OA) [26].

The lncRNA HOTTIP, encoded in the HOXA cluster, was shown to play a crucial role in the persistent activation of myofibroblasts promoting chronic inflammation and collagen deposition [53]. Silencing of HOTTIP reduced inflammation in a mouse model of arthritis and modified synovial fibroblast function by DNA demethylation of the locus encoding SFRP1 (Secreted Frizzled Related Protein 1), a modulator of the Wnt signaling pathway [54].

5.3 Gastrointestinal fibroblasts

The adult gastrointestinal tract was shown to keep the position-specific expression pattern of HOX genes along the anteroposterior axis of embryonic development, recapitulating the expression pattern in the embryonic gastrointestinal tract [55]. HOX gene expression varied over 11 different measured gastrointestinal sites and clearly separated segments of the upper gastrointestinal tract from segments of the lower gastrointestinal tract. Accordingly, differences in HOX gene expression were found by comparing the gene expression profile of gastrointestinal fibroblasts isolated from the stomach, ileum and the colon. In particular, HOX paralogs with lower numbers (e.g. *HOXA2*, *HOXD3*) were preferentially expressed in the esophagus and stomach, while HOX paralogues with higher numbers (e.g. *HOXA10*, *HOXD10*) tended to be more expressed in the cecum and rectum. Using hierarchical clustering analysis, different subgroups of gastrointestinal fibroblasts were identified based on differences in transcriptional regulation, signaling ligands, and extracellular matrix remodeling [56].

Gastrointestinal fibroblasts play a pivotal role in gastrointestinal epithelial renewal by supporting epithelial cell differentiation, and they have been described to contribute to gastrointestinal inflammation and fibrosis [57, 58]. Furthermore, gastrointestinal fibroblasts are strongly involved in the initiation, progression and metastasis of gastrointestinal cancer [59]. For instance, increased expression of HOXA13, *HOXB13* and *HOXC13* was found in esophageal pathologies such as esophageal squamous cell cancer, Barrett's esophagus or esophageal adenocarcinoma [60, 61]. Aberrant expression these HOX paralogues, which are normally less expressed in upper gastrointestinal parts might contribute to the activation of pathogenic processes at this site. Together these observations suggest that HOX genes might play a role in steering position-specific processes during gut inflammation and cancer development [62]. Unfortunately, up to know functional studies are lacking that analyzed the impact of site-specific HOX expression on gut homeostasis and disease development.

6. HOX genes in hematopoietic cells

Apart from stromal cells, HOX genes are expressed in hematopoietic stem cells and progenitors in early development, with a pattern characteristic of the lineage and stage of differentiation of the cell. Using gene targeting technology and gain-of-function and loss-of-function mutations, the function of HOX genes in hematopoiesis has been extensively investigated [63].

For example, HOXB3, HOXB4 and HOXA9 are highly expressed in uncommitted hematopoietic cells, whereas HOXB8 and HOXA10 are expressed in myeloid committed cells. The different HOX clusters also have specific patterns of lineage-restricted expression, whereby HOXA genes are expressed in myeloid cells, HOXB genes in erythroid cells and HOXC genes in lymphoid cells. Intriguingly, the HOXD genes are not expressed in hematopoiesis despite having similar regulatory regions to the other clusters [64–66].

These observations indicate that modulation of the expression of a particular HOX gene can alter cell phenotype and suggest a causal relationship for lineage-specific patterns of HOX gene expression [67].

7. HOX genes in disease

7.1 HOX genes in cardiovascular disease

Steadily increasing evidence supports the idea that gene expression diversities in the vascular system are a major contributing factor in determining region-specific cardiovascular disease susceptibility. The regionally distinct and topographic expression patterns of HOX transcription factors in embryonic development is remembered in vascular smooth muscle cells [68] as well as in endothelial cells [7, 18, 69]. The persistent topographic expression patterns in post-natal vascular tissues suggest that HOX genes play a critical role in maintaining vessel wall homeostasis in a region-specific manner [70]. Intriguingly, in adult mice, high-throughput mRNA profiling revealed that HOX paralogues 6-10 (Hox6-10) are higher expressed in the thoracic aorta, which is resistant to atherosclerotic lesions, than in the aortic arch, which is highly athero-susceptible [68]. In humans, the differential expression of HOXA9 gene contributed to phenotypic differences in smooth muscle cells from athero-resistant compared athero-susceptible regions, which might be connected to the site-specific development of atherosclerotic plaques. For example, region-specific reciprocal interactions of HOXA9 with the pro-inflammatory transcription factor NF-κB have been demonstrated. In general, genetic regulatory networks of cardiovascular diseases processes implicated genes of various functional categories such as ECM remodeling, transmembrane signaling, cell cycle control, and inflammatory response as potentially HOX-dependent.

Ectopic activation of HOXC10 and HOXC9 in atherosclerotic coronary arteries has been found to be associated with loss of DNA methylation within the HOXC11/HOXC9 genomic interval [34, 71]. These data define epigenetic mechanisms controlling HOX expression as critical in aberrant expression of HOX and HOX-target genes in cardiovascular disease [72].

7.2 HOX genes in solid cancers

In embryogenesis, a fine balance between cell proliferation and differentiation is essential for normal development of the fetus, but in cancer, the balance between the two processes is impaired [63, 73].

Studies suggest that the expression of HOX genes becomes dysregulated during development of various solid tumors, including colon, breast, prostate, lung, glioblastomas, thyroid, bladder, ovarian, melanoma, and kidney cancers [74, 75]. In fact, the specific pattern of change in HOX gene expression is dependent on cancer type, tumor stage, and, in certain cases, on anatomic location [76].

HOX genes have been identified to be important regulators of cancer stem cells (CSCs) which are critical for initiation and progression of solid tumors [33, 74]. These genes act as transcriptional activators as well as transcriptional repressors in cancers [77]. Studies show that the expression of specific HOX genes in cancers tends to differ based on tissue type and tumor site. HOXA genes were often reported to have altered expression in breast and ovarian cancers, HOXB genes in colon cancers, HOXC genes in prostate and lung cancer and HOXD genes in colon and breast cancers. This pattern can be linked to the embryonic origin of tissues. For example, colon, prostate, and lung, originating from endodermal, showed relatively similar HOXA and HOXB family gene expression patterns compared to breast tumors arising from mammary tissue, which originates from the ectoderm [74].

The differential expression of HOX genes in various solid tumors provides an opportunity to advance our understanding of cancer development and to develop new therapeutic agents. Specific methylation profiles in HOX clusters or in HOX-associated histones are recognized as potential biomarkers in several cancers and can be exploited in cancer therapy. The use of epigenetic drugs affecting generalized or specific DNA methylation profiles is a promising approach in cancer therapy in the near future. However, since the generalized effect of epigenetic drugs may lead to secondary malignancies, the development of drugs targeting specific epigenetic alterations, including those related to HOX genes, could advance this therapeutic approach [78].

HOX genes are recognized as potential therapeutic targets in adrenocortical tumors. Understanding the pathway being regulated by the transcription factor HOXB9, which promotes adrenal tumor progression through an increase in the expression of cell cycle genes, including Ccne1, could help to development potential drug targets for adrenocortical carcinoma [79]. Moreover, HOX peptide inhibitor showed a promising effect on cell survival in mice and could be used as peptide-based cancer therapeutics [80].

Analyses of HOX gene expression in normal breast tissue and primary breast cancers [81] showed that several HOX genes are differentially expressed in breast cancer compared to normal breast tissues, with different breast cancer tissues and cell lines showing high variability in the pattern of HOX gene expression [81]. Thus, these studies support the idea that aberrant expression of HOX genes is involved in the development of breast cancer and in the malignant behavior of cancer cells, but shows that, at least in breast cancer, there is no uniform pattern of HOX gene alterations that lead to malignant growth of cells.

The stroma surrounding solid tumors is built from cancer-associated fibroblasts (CAFs) which are recognized to play a significant role in tumor growth. Interestingly, it could be shown that CAFs predominantly develop from local fibroblasts at the site of the tumor [82]. Therefore, site-specific differences in local fibroblasts surrounding the tumor might be crucially involved in tumor development and invasiveness. Furthermore, site-specific differences in fibroblasts might be connected to the site-specific distribution of cancer metastases in certain organs [83]. This would support the “seed and soil” hypothesis, which states that the distribution pattern of metastases is highly dependent on the microenvironment of the organ in which the metastases are located [84]. Unfortunately, an analysis of the expression and influence of HOX genes in CAFs from different tumor sites is missing up to now.

7.3 HOX genes in joint and bone disease

Mammalian HOX genes are critical for proper development of skeletal morphology during embryogenesis. The continuous function of HOX genes in the skeleton after the establishment of skeletal morphology has been determined using genetic tools in mouse models [85]. The generation of a conditional Hoxd11 allele that can be deleted at adult stages after normal development and growth of the skeleton was used to show that Hox genes in the adult skeleton regulate the differentiation of skeletal stem cells into bone cells [86]. These data convincingly showed that Hox gene function in the skeleton is not restricted to development and that Hox genes play a crucial, functional role in adult bone homeostasis.

Furthermore, functional importance of Hox genes in the regulation of chondrocyte differentiation has been demonstrated [85, 87]. Hox genes are involved in the regulation of the progression of cells along the chondrogenic differentiation pathway after the initial formation of the cartilage anlagen. However, overexpression of a Hoxc8 transgene caused cartilage defects whose severity depended on the dosage of the transgene [85]. The abnormal cartilage was characterized by an accumulation of proliferating chondrocytes and reduced maturation. These results suggest that Hoxc8 continues to regulate cartilage homeostasis after development, presumably by controlling the progression of cells along the chondrocyte differentiation pathway. Their capacity for regulation of cartilage differentiation suggests that HOX genes could also be involved in human chondrodysplasias or other cartilage disorders [85].

Arthritic joints are characterized by rearrangements and dysregulated gene expression of bone, cartilage and synovial tissues [88, 89]. The exact molecular and cellular events leading to the development of the different kinds of arthritis still remain elusive, but involvement of HOX gene regulation in the key tissues affected by rheumatic muscular-skeletal diseases indicate a potential link between arthritis development and HOX transcription factors. HOX genes were for instance associated with the onset and development of osteoarthritis (OA) (e.g. HOXA9 in hip OA) and as mentioned above with pathogenic important joint-specific functions of synovial fibroblasts in RA [45, 90, 91]. However, it has not been clarified up to know whether changes of expression of HOX genes in OA are specific for a specific joint region or a common feature of disease.

Like a number of human diseases, rheumatic diseases include characteristic pathologies in specific anatomical locations [21, 44]. For example, ankylosing spondylitis is a chronic inflammatory disease affecting the spinal vertebrae and sacroiliac joints, causing debilitating pain and loss of mobility [92]. Joints in the hands, are commonly involved in RA and OA [93]. Reactive arthritis is a rheumatic condition that causes inflammation particularly in knees [94]. Several mechanisms might be involved in this susceptibility of specific joints for developing specific forms of arthritis. In addition to and maybe in combination with local mechanic factors, site-specific gene expression of local cell types (bone, cartilage, synovium), potentially regulated by HOX genes, might be crucially involved in the development of specific arthritides in specific joint locations. Furthermore, disease-specific systemic triggers, such as specific auto-antibodies or cytokines might preferentially affect local cell types at a specific anatomic sites [95].

8. Conclusions

HOX genes, a family of homeodomain transcription factors, guide embryonic development by encoding positional information during axis formation, determining site specificity of the body plan and regulating formation of structures along the various body axes.

Like other transcription factors, HOX genes control the establishment and maintenance of specific cell states by regulating distinct sets of downstream genes. Despite their similar DNA-binding properties, they have highly specific effects on the transcriptome. This genetic control results in functional diversity of various body parts. Cells such as fibroblasts thus develop not only an organ-specific but also a site-specific transcriptional program. Intriguingly, these HOX regulated transcriptional programs are epigenetically maintained in adult cells.

Several studies endorse that regulation of site-specific gene expression by HOX genes contribute to the development of a broad range of diseases (**Figure 2**). The site-specific environment created by the expression of specific HOX genes might promote or prevent the development of diseases at specific locations, in line with

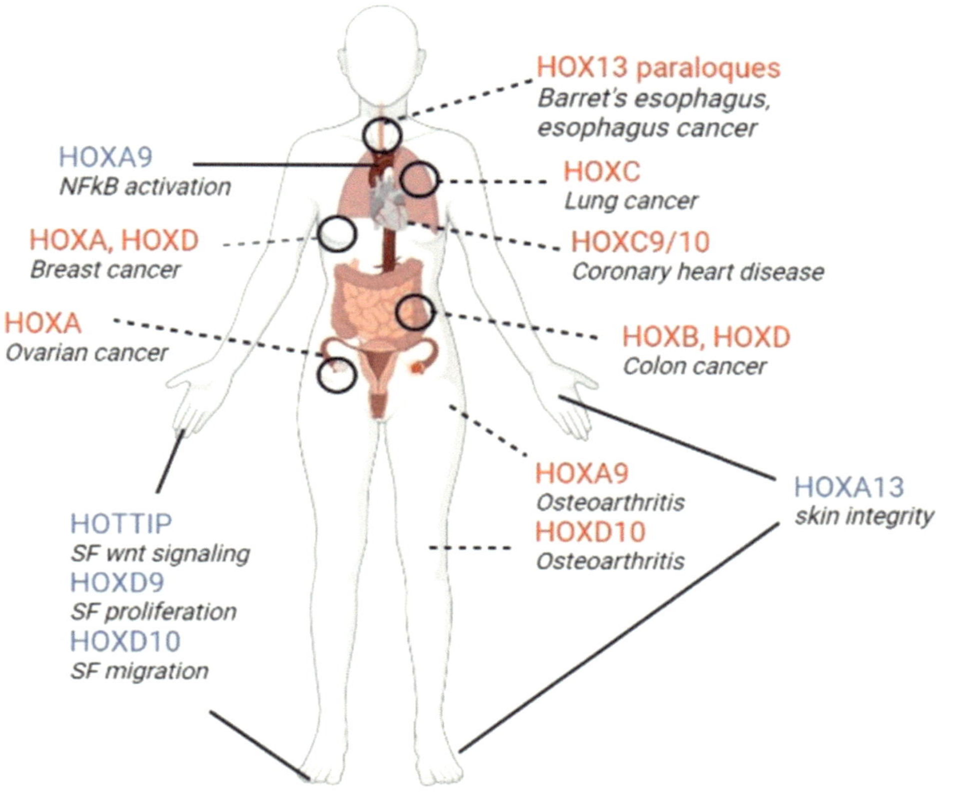

Figure 2.
Summary of diseases that have been associated with HOX gene expression. In some cases (blue letters) regular site-specific expression of HOX genes has been connected to disease development based on the functions of the respective HOX genes (below in italics). In other cases, aberrant expression of HOX genes (red letters) was associated with the development of diseases (below in italics). SF = synovial fibroblasts. The figure was created with Biorender.

the 'seed and soil' hypothesis. Furthermore, activation or repression of HOX expression during disease development, potentially by modulation of the epigenetic mechanisms regulating the HOX loci, might further influence site-specific disease processes.

Therefore, a better understanding of site-specific cellular and molecular mechanisms underlying regional appearance of disease is essential for understanding disease development and designing new therapeutic approaches.

Conflict of interest

The authors declare no conflict of interest.

Author details

Masoumeh Mirrahimi and Caroline Ospelt*
Center of Experimental Rheumatology, Department of Rheumatology, University Hospital of Zurich, University of Zurich, Switzerland

*Address all correspondence to: caroline.ospelt@usz.ch

References

[1] Iimura T, Denans N, Pourquié OJCtidb. Establishment of Hox vertebral identities in the embryonic spine precursors. 2009;88:201-234.

[2] Konttinen YT, Li T-F, Hukkanen M, Ma J, Xu J-W, Virtanen IJAR, et al. Fibroblast biology Signals targeting the synovial fibroblast in arthritis. 2000; 2(5):1-8.

[3] Miller MA, Zachary JFJPbovd. Mechanisms and morphology of cellular injury, adaptation, and death. 2017:2.

[4] Foote AG, Wang Z, Kendziorski C, Thibeault SLJBg. Tissue specific human fibroblast differential expression based on RNAsequencing analysis. 2019;20(1): 1-19.

[5] Dickmeis T, Müller FJBiFG. The identification and functional characterisation of conserved regulatory elements in developmental genes. 2005;3(4):332-350.

[6] Sonawane AR, Platig J, Fagny M, Chen C-Y, Paulson JN, Lopes-Ramos CM, et al. Understanding tissue-specific gene regulation. 2017;21(4):1077-1088.

[7] Chang HY, Chi J-T, Dudoit S, Bondre C, van de Rijn M, Botstein D, et al. Diversity, topographic differentiation, and positional memory in human fibroblasts. 2002;99(20): 12877-12882.

[8] Hueber SD, Lohmann IJB. Shaping segments: Hox gene function in the genomic age. 2008;30(10):965-979.

[9] Baker CV, Bronner-Fraser MJDb. Vertebrate cranial placodes I. Embryonic induction. 2001;232(1):1-61.

[10] Füchtbauer EM, Westphal HJDd. MyoD and myogenin are coexpressed in regenerating skeletal muscle of the mouse. 1992;193(1):34-39.

[11] Prouty SM, Lawrence L, Stenn KJLi, methods ajot, pathology. Fibroblast-dependent induction of a murine skin lesion similar to human nevus sebaceus of Jadassohn. 1997;76(2):179-189.

[12] Yamaguchi Y, Itami S, Tarutani M, Hosokawa K, Miura H, Yoshikawa KJJoid. Regulation of keratin 9 in nonpalmoplantar keratinocytes by palmoplantar fibroblasts through epithelial–mesenchymal interactions. 1999;112(4):483-8.

[13] Ferrier DEJFiE, Evolution. Evolution of homeobox gene clusters in animals: the giga-cluster and primary vs. secondary clustering. 2016;4:36.

[14] Luo Z, Rhie SK, Farnham PJJC. The enigmatic hox genes: Can we crack their code? 2019;11(3):323.

[15] Svingen T, Tonissen KJH. Hox transcription factors and their elusive mammalian gene targets. 2006;97(2): 88-96.

[16] Furukubo-Tokunaga K, Flister S, Gehring WJJPotNAoS. Functional specificity of the Antennapedia homeodomain. 1993;90(13):6360-6364.

[17] Chan S-K, Jaffe L, Capovilla M, Botas J, Mann RSJC. The DNA binding specificity of Ultrabithorax is modulated by cooperative interactions with extradenticle, another homeoprotein. 1994;78(4):603-615.

[18] Rinn JL, Bondre C, Gladstone HB, Brown PO, Chang HYJPG. Anatomic demarcation by positional variation in fibroblast gene expression programs. 2006;2(7):e119.

[19] McClintock JM, Carlson R, Mann DM, Prince VEJD. Consequences of Hox gene duplication in the vertebrates: an investigation of the zebrafish Hox paralogue group 1 genes. 2001;128(13):2471-84.

[20] Krumlauf RJC. Hox genes in vertebrate development. 1994;78(2): 191-201.

[21] Tabin CJJD. Why we have (only) five fingers per hand: Hox genes and the evolution of paired limbs. 1992;116(2): 289-96.

[22] Goodman F, Scambler PJCg. Human HOX gene mutations. 2001;59(1):1-11.

[23] Noordermeer D, Leleu M, Schorderet P, Joye E, Chabaud F, Duboule DJe. Temporal dynamics and developmental memory of 3D chromatin architecture at Hox gene loci. 2014;3:e02557.

[24] Zákány J, Duboule DJN. Synpolydactyly in mice with a targeted deficiency in the HoxD complex. 1996;384(6604):69-71.

[25] Williams TM, Williams ME, Kuick R, Misek D, McDonagh K, Hanash S, et al. Candidate downstream regulated genes of HOX group 13 transcription factors with and without monomeric DNA binding capability. 2005;279(2):462-80.

[26] Luan L, Ma Y, Zhang LJE, medicine t. HOXD10 silencing suppresses human fibroblast-like synoviocyte migration in rheumatoid arthritis via downregulation of the p38/JNK pathway. 2018;16(3): 1621-8.

[27] Knosp WM, Scott V, Bächinger HP, Stadler HS. HOXA13 regulates the expression of bone morphogenetic proteins 2 and 7 to control distal limb morphogenesis. 2004.

[28] Praggastis SA, Thummel CSJG, development. Right time, right place: the temporal regulation of developmental gene expression. 2017;31(9):847-848.

[29] Soshnikova N, Duboule DJE. Epigenetic regulation of vertebrate Hox genes: a dynamic equilibrium. 2009;4(8):537-540.

[30] Shahhoseini M, Taghizadeh Z, Hatami M, Baharvand HJB, Biology C. Retinoic acid dependent histone 3 demethylation of the clustered HOX genes during neural differentiation of human embryonic stem cells. 2013;91(2):116-22.

[31] Bernstein BE, Mikkelsen TS, Xie X, Kamal M, Huebert DJ, Cuff J, et al. A bivalent chromatin structure marks key developmental genes in embryonic stem cells. 2006;125(2):315-326.

[32] Kojima T, Takahashi NJCA-CS, Mechanisms. Hox genes and teratogenic factors. 2012.

[33] Seifert A, Werheid DF, Knapp SM, Tobiasch EJWjosc. Role of Hox genes in stem cell differentiation. 2015;7(3):583.

[34] Tsumagari K, Baribault C, Terragni J, Chandra S, Renshaw C, Sun Z, et al. DNA methylation and differentiation: HOX genes in muscle cells. 2013;6(1):1-17.

[35] Statello L, Guo C-J, Chen L-L, Huarte MJNRMCB. Gene regulation by long non-coding RNAs and its biological functions. 2021;22(2):96-118.

[36] Zhang X, Wang W, Zhu W, Dong J, Cheng Y, Yin Z, et al. Mechanisms and functions of long non-coding RNAs at multiple regulatory levels. 2019; 20(22):5573.

[37] Heubach J, Monsior J, Deenen R, Niegisch G, Szarvas T, Niedworok C, et al. The long noncoding RNA HOTAIR has tissue and cell type-dependent effects on HOX gene expression and phenotype of urothelial cancer cells. 2015;14(1):1-17.

[38] Selleri L, Bartolomei MS, Bickmore WA, He L, Stubbs L, Reik W, et al. A Hox-embedded long noncoding

RNA: is it all hot air? 2016;12(12): e1006485.

[39] Wang KC, Yang YW, Liu B, Sanyal A, Corces-Zimmerman R, Chen Y, et al. A long noncoding RNA maintains active chromatin to coordinate homeotic gene expression. 2011;472(7341):120-124.

[40] He H, Hua X, Yan JJO. Epigenetic regulations in hematopoietic Hox code. 2011;30(4):379-388.

[41] Rinn JL, Wang JK, Allen N, Brugmann SA, Mikels AJ, Liu H, et al. A dermal HOX transcriptional program regulates site-specific epidermal fate. Genes & development. 2008;22(3): 303-307.

[42] Fu DJ, Thomson C, Lunny DP, Dopping-Hepenstal PJ, McGrath JA, Smith FJD, et al. Keratin 9 is required for the structural integrity and terminal differentiation of the palmoplantar epidermis. J Invest Dermatol. 2014;134(3):754-763.

[43] Ospelt C. Synovial fibroblasts in 2017. RMD Open. 2017;3(2):e000471.

[44] Frank-Bertoncelj M, Trenkmann M, Klein K, Karouzakis E, Rehrauer H, Bratus A, et al. Epigenetically-driven anatomical diversity of synovial fibroblasts guides joint-specific fibroblast functions. 2017;8(1):1-14.

[45] Ai R, Hammaker D, Boyle DL, Morgan R, Walsh AM, Fan S, et al. Joint-specific DNA methylation and transcriptome signatures in rheumatoid arthritis identify distinct pathogenic processes. 2016;7(1):1-9.

[46] Chau NN, Hirose T, Nakazawa M, Kobata T, Nakamura H, Nishioka K, et al. Expression of HOXD9 in fibroblast-like synoviocytes from rheumatoid arthritis patients. 2002;10(1):41-8.

[47] Montavon T, Soshnikova N, editors. Hox gene regulation and timing in embryogenesis. Seminars in cell & developmental biology; 2014: Elsevier.

[48] Zakany J, Duboule DJCoig, development. The role of Hox genes during vertebrate limb development. 2007;17(4):359-366.

[49] Xue C, Hasunuma T, Asahara H, Yin W, Maeda T, Fujisawa K, et al. Transcriptional regulation of the HOX4C gene by basic fibroblast growth factor on rheumatoid synovial fibroblasts. 1997;40(9):1628-35.

[50] Rinn JL, Kertesz M, Wang JK, Squazzo SL, Xu X, Brugmann SA, et al. Functional demarcation of active and silent chromatin domains in human HOX loci by noncoding RNAs. 2007;129(7):1311-1323.

[51] Hung T, Chang HYJRb. Long noncoding RNA in genome regulation: prospects and mechanisms. 2010;7(5):582-585.

[52] Karouzakis E, Gay RE, Michel BA, Gay S, Neidhart MJA, Rheumatology ROJotACo. DNA hypomethylation in rheumatoid arthritis synovial fibroblasts. 2009;60(12):3613-3622.

[53] Lee Y-H, Yu C-C, Hsieh P-L, Liao Y-W, Yu C-H, Su T-RJJotFMA. Inhibition of lncRNA HOTTIP ameliorated myofibroblast activities and inflammatory cytokines in oral submucous fibrosis. 2021;120(5): 1188-1193.

[54] Hu X, Tang J, Hu X, Bao P, Deng W, Wu J, et al. Silencing of long non-coding RNA HOTTIP reduces inflammation in rheumatoid arthritis by demethylation of SFRP1. 2020;19:468-481.

[55] Yahagi N, Kosaki R, Ito T, Mitsuhashi T, Shimada H, Tomita M, et al. Position-specific expression of Hox genes along the gastrointestinal tract. Congenit Anom (Kyoto). 2004;44(1): 18-26.

[56] Higuchi Y, Kojima M, Ishii G, Aoyagi K, Sasaki H, Ochiai AJPO. Gastrointestinal fibroblasts have specialized, diverse transcriptional phenotypes: a comprehensive gene expression analysis of human fibroblasts. 2015;10(6):e0129241.

[57] Andoh A, Bamba S, Brittan M, Fujiyama Y, Wright NA. Role of intestinal subepithelial myofibroblasts in inflammation and regenerative response in the gut. Pharmacol Ther. 2007;114(1):94-106.

[58] Rieder F, Fiocchi C. Intestinal fibrosis in inflammatory bowel disease - Current knowledge and future perspectives. J Crohns Colitis. 2008;2(4):279-290.

[59] Dang H, Harryvan TJ, Hawinkels L. Fibroblast Subsets in Intestinal Homeostasis, Carcinogenesis, Tumor Progression, and Metastasis. Cancers (Basel). 2021;13(2).

[60] Takahashi O, Hamada J-i, Abe M, Hata S, Asano T, Takahashi Y, et al. Dysregulated expression of HOX and ParaHOX genes in human esophageal squamous cell carcinoma. 2007;17(4):753-760.

[61] Gu Z-D, Shen L-Y, Wang H, Chen X-M, Li Y, Ning T, et al. HOXA13 promotes cancer cell growth and predicts poor survival of patients with esophageal squamous cell carcinoma. 2009;69(12):4969-73.

[62] Calon A, Gross I, Lhermitte B, Martin E, Beck F, Duclos B, et al. Different effects of the Cdx1 and Cdx2 homeobox genes in a murine model of intestinal inflammation. 2007;56(12):1688-95.

[63] Grier D, Thompson A, Kwasniewska A, McGonigle G, Halliday H, Lappin TJTJoPAJotPSoGB, et al. The pathophysiology of HOX genes and their role in cancer. 2005;205(2):154-171.

[64] Giampaolo A, Sterpetti P, Bulgarini D, Samoggia P, Pelosi E, Valtieri M, et al. Key functional role and lineage-specific expression of selected HOXB genes in purified hematopoietic progenitor differentiation. 1994.

[65] Kawagoe H, Humphries R, Blair A, Sutherland H, Hogge DJL. Expression of HOX genes, HOX cofactors, and MLL in phenotypically and functionally defined subpopulations of leukemic and normal human hematopoietic cells. 1999; 13(5):687-698.

[66] Pineault N, Helgason CD, Lawrence HJ, Humphries RKJEh. Differential expression of Hox, Meis1, and Pbx1 genes in primitive cells throughout murine hematopoietic ontogeny. 2002;30(1):49-57.

[67] Alharbi RA, Pettengell R, Pandha HS, Morgan RJL. The role of HOX genes in normal hematopoiesis and acute leukemia. 2013;27(5): 1000-1008.

[68] Trigueros-Motos L, González-Granado JM, Cheung C, Fernández P, Sánchez-Cabo F, Dopazo A, et al. Embryological-origin–dependent differences in homeobox expression in adult aorta: role in regional phenotypic variability and regulation of NF-κB activity. 2013;33(6):1248-1256.

[69] Wang KC, Helms JA, Chang HYJTicb. Regeneration, repair and remembering identity: the three Rs of Hox gene expression. 2009;19(6): 268-275.

[70] Visconti RP, Awgulewitsch AJWjobc. Topographic patterns of vascular disease: HOX proteins as determining factors? 2015;6(3):65.

[71] Tickle C. The Hox gene network in vertebrate limb development. HOX Gene Expression: Springer; 2007. p. 42-52.

[72] Castillo-Díaz SA, Garay-Sevilla ME, Hernández-González MA, Solís-Martínez MO, Zaina SJIjomm. Extensive demethylation of normally hypermethylated CpG islands occurs in human atherosclerotic arteries. 2010;26(5):691-700.

[73] Lappin TR, Grier DG, Thompson A, Halliday HLJTUmj. HOX genes: seductive science, mysterious mechanisms. 2006;75(1):23.

[74] Bhatlekar S, Fields JZ, Boman BMJJomm. HOX genes and their role in the development of human cancers. 2014;92(8):811-823.

[75] Li L, Wang Y, Song G, Zhang X, Gao S, Liu HJCl. HOX cluster-embedded antisense long non-coding RNAs in lung cancer. 2019;450:14-21.

[76] López-Romero R, Marrero-Rodríguez D, Romero-Morelos P, Villegas V, Valdivia A, Arreola H, et al. The role of developmental HOX genes in cervical cancer. 2015;53:S188.

[77] Li B, Huang Q, Wei G-HJC. The role of HOX transcription factors in cancer predisposition and progression. 2019;11(4):528.

[78] Paço A, de Bessa Garcia SA, Freitas RJC. Methylation in HOX clusters and its applications in cancer therapy. 2020;9(7):1613.

[79] Francis JC, Gardiner JR, Renaud Y, Chauhan R, Weinstein Y, Gomez-Sanchez C, et al. HOX genes promote cell proliferation and are potential therapeutic targets in adrenocortical tumours. 2021;124(4): 805-816.

[80] Xiao Y-F, Jie M-M, Li B-S, Hu C-J, Xie R, Tang B, et al. Peptide-based treatment: a promising cancer therapy. 2015;2015.

[81] Costa BM, Smith JS, Chen Y, Chen J, Phillips HS, Aldape KD, et al. Reversing HOXA9 oncogene activation by PI3K inhibition: epigenetic mechanism and prognostic significance in human glioblastoma. 2010;70(2):453-62.

[82] Arina A, Idel C, Hyjek EM, Alegre M-L, Wang Y, Bindokas VP, et al. Tumor-associated fibroblasts predominantly come from local and not circulating precursors. 2016;113(27): 7551-7556.

[83] Klein-Goldberg A, Maman S, Witz IPJCl. The role played by the microenvironment in site-specific metastasis. 2014;352(1):54-58.

[84] Fidler IJ, Poste GJTlo. The "seed and soil" hypothesis revisited. 2008;9(8): 808.

[85] Yueh YG, Gardner DP, Kappen CJPotNAoS. Evidence for regulation of cartilage differentiation by the homeobox gene Hoxc-8. 1998; 95(17):9956-61.

[86] Song JY, Pineault KM, Dones JM, Raines RT, Wellik DMJPotNAoS. Hox genes maintain critical roles in the adult skeleton. 2020;117(13):7296-7304.

[87] Gross S, Krause Y, Wuelling M, Vortkamp AJPo. Hoxa11 and Hoxd11 regulate chondrocyte differentiation upstream of Runx2 and Shox2 in mice. 2012;7(8):e43553.

[88] Chen Y-J, Chang W-A, Wu L-Y, Huang C-F, Chen C-H, Kuo P-LJIjoms. Identification of novel genes in osteoarthritic fibroblast-like synoviocytes using next-generation sequencing and bioinformatics approaches. 2019;16(8):1057.

[89] Thysen S, Luyten FP, Lories RJJDm, mechanisms. Targets, models and challenges in osteoarthritis research. 2015;8(1):17-30.

[90] Delgado-Calle J, Fernández AF, Sainz J, Zarrabeitia MT, Sañudo C, García-Renedo R, et al. Genome-wide profiling of bone reveals differentially methylated regions in osteoporosis and osteoarthritis. 2013;65(1):197-205.

[91] Pelttari K, Barbero A, Martin IJAotm. A potential role of homeobox transcription factors in osteoarthritis. 2015;3(17).

[92] Ghasemi-Rad M, Attaya H, Lesha E, Vegh A, Maleki-Miandoab T, Nosair E, et al. Ankylosing spondylitis: A state of the art factual backbone. 2015;7(9):236.

[93] Ospelt C, Frank-Bertoncelj MJNRR. Why location matters—site-specific factors in rheumatic diseases. 2017;13(7):433-442.

[94] Carter JD, Hudson APJRDC. Reactive arthritis: clinical aspects and medical management. 2009;35(1):21-44.

[95] Theofilopoulos AN, Kono DH, Baccala RJNi. The multiple pathways to autoimmunity. 2017;18(7):716-724.

Chapter 2

Mesenchymal Stem/Stromal Cells and Fibroblasts: Their Roles in Tissue Injury and Regeneration, and Age-Related Degeneration

Janja Zupan

Abstract

Mesenchymal stem/stromal cells (MSCs) and fibroblasts are present in normal tissues to support tissue homeostasis. Both share common pathways and have a number of common features, such as a spindle-shaped morphology, connective tissue localization, and multipotency. In inflammation, a nonspecific response to injury, fibroblasts and MSC are the main players. Two mechanisms of their mode of action have been defined: immunomodulation and regeneration. Following tissue injury, MSCs are activated, and they multiply and differentiate, to mitigate the damage. With aging and, in particular, in degenerative disorders of the musculoskeletal system (i.e., joint and bone disorders), the regenerative capacity of MSCs appears to be lost or diverted into the production of other nonfunctional cell types, such as adipocytes and fibroblasts. Fibroblasts are stromal cells that provide the majority of the structural framework of almost all types of tissues; i.e., the stroma. As such, fibroblasts also have significant roles in tissue development, maintenance, and repair. In their immunosuppressive role, MSCs and fibroblasts contribute to the normal resolution of inflammation that is a prerequisite for successful tissue repair. In this chapter, we review the common and opposing properties of different tissue-derived MSCs and fibroblasts under physiological and pathophysiological conditions. We consider injury and age-related degeneration of various tissues, and also some immunological disorders. Specifically, we address the distinct and common features of both cell types in health and disease, with a focus on human synovial joints. Finally, we also discuss the possible approaches to boost the complementary roles of MSCs and fibroblasts, to promote successful tissue regeneration.

Keywords: Mesenchymal stem/stromal cells, fibroblasts, tissue injury, age-related tissue degeneration, tissue regeneration

1. Introduction

Mesenchymal stem/stromal cells (MSCs) represent tissue-resident progenitor cells with multi-differentiation potential *in vivo* (stem cells) and *in vitro* (stromal cells) [1]. Although MSCs were first described several decades ago [2, 3], their nature, roles, definitions, and even name remain to be fully defined. The largest bone of contention lies in their designation as stem cells. Even Arnold Caplan, who first coined the term 'mesenchymal stem cells' [4], has suggested recently that it is time to change the name, to avoid unprecedented expectations of regrowth of new tissues and organs [5]. About 15 years ago, the International Society for Cellular Therapy set up minimal criteria for the definition of MSCs *in vitro*, which include plastic adherence, trilineage differentiation, and a set of negative and positive markers [6]. These initial efforts were further up-graded as the knowledge of the *in-vitro* properties of MSCs accumulated, in particular for their role in immunomodulation [7].

Great advances have been made in the *in-vivo* identification of human skeletal stem cells (SSCs). Following their identification in mouse bone marrow, Chan et al. unraveled the hierarchy of positive markers (i.e., podoplanin, CD73, CD164) and negative markers (i.e., CD146) of the self-renewing, multipotent human SSCs. These cells can be isolated from human fetal and adult adipose stroma following treatment with bone morphogenetic protein 2, and they can undergo local expansion in response to acute skeletal injury [8]. In addition, the same group recently identified a way to boost the endogenous SSCs to aid in the repair of worn out cartilage in osteoarthritis [9].

In contrast to the huge advances made in the field of bone-marrow-derived MSCs, the identity and role of MSCs resident in other tissues are still largely unknown. Initially, MSCs were believed to be common progenitors of all musculoskeletal tissues. On this basis, several hypotheses on the developmental origins of MSCs were put forward. The pericyte hypothesis, for example, suggested that MSCs are pericytes and are thus common to every vascularized tissue [10]. However, Guimarães-Camboa et al. rejected this theory, and revealed that pericytes do not behave as stem cells during aging and injury [11]. They traced transcription factor Tbx18 (as a selective marker of pericytes and vascular smooth muscle cells) to follow the fate of these cells in aging and in injury models in multiple adult organs. In this way they showed that pericytes maintained their identity through aging and in diverse pathological settings, and hence did not significantly contribute to other cell lineages [11]. Currently, what we do know is that MSCs are tissue-specific progenitors that can differentiate into their tissue of origin [12, 13] and exhibit tissue of origin-specific profiles and response to inflammatory stimuli [14]. Although MSCs have already been used in clinical practice in the form of cell injections for treatment of several degenerative disorders, unfortunately much of their reported anti-aging and regenerative potential remains unsupported [15, 16]. Hence, their potential in regenerative medicine is still largely underexploited.

Fibroblasts are historically even 'older' than MSCs, as they were first described over a century ago [17]. However the criteria for their definition is even more poorly established than that for MSCs [18–20]. Fibroblasts constitute the majority of the cells of the structural framework, or stroma, of almost all types of tissues [20]. Their main role is the secretion of extracellular matrix molecules, such as collagen, proteoglycans, and others. As the different types of collagen are the major component of tissues such as bone, cartilage, and skin, fibroblasts also have significant roles in tissue development, maintenance, and repair. Fibroblasts from different tissues were long considered as functionally homogenous cells, however significant differences in transcriptome, epigenome and function were demonstrated for synovial fibroblasts from different anatomical locations in joints [21]. Under certain conditions, fibroblasts can also transform into more aggressive phenotypes and contribute to disease pathophysiology, such as in cancers and rheumatoid arthritis [22].

Mesenchymal stem/stromal cells and fibroblasts share numerous common features, as has been reviewed elsewhere [20, 23]. As these cells participate in the common pathways of tissue development, maintenance and healing, either working together or in opposition, this chapter provides an overview of recent studies on these shared and opposing properties of MSCs and fibroblasts with a focus on tissue injury and age-related tissue degeneration, in particular in joint health and disease.

For the purpose of this review, we performed a literature search in PubMed according to the search terms and filters shown in **Figure 1**. To focus on human studies carried out in the past 5 years, we excluded all studies dealing with tumor

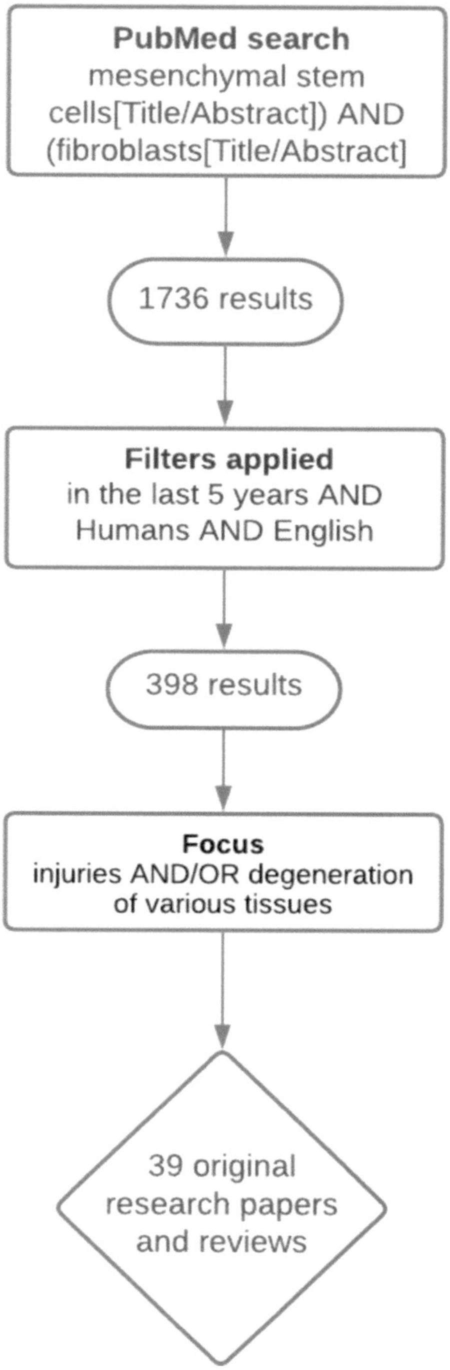

Figure 1.
The approach used to search and select the papers included in this review.

research, which covers a particularly large research area. We included only those studies dealing with tissue injuries and regeneration, and age-related degeneration. Finally, we also discuss the options for diverting tissue healing processes toward morphological and functional regeneration, rather than the creation of poorly functioning scar tissue to cover such defects.

2. MSCs and fibroblasts in general: their common and distinct properties

A summary of the recent studies that have compared various tissue-derived MSCs and fibroblasts face to face is provided in **Table 1**. A schematic representation of the distinct and common features of MSCs and fibroblasts in health and disease, with a focus on human synovial joints is shown in **Figure 2**.

Reference	Source of MSCs	Source of fibroblasts	Methods	Findings
[24]	MSCs (Lonza)	Normal dermis	Inflammatory stimulation and subsequent treatment with dexamethasone; multidimensional molecular profiling	Induction of the secretion of cytokines, proteases, and other inflammation agonists and pro- and anti-inflammatory eicosanoids; dexamethasone down-regulated most cytokines and proteases, and pro- and anti-inflammatory eicosanoids; similar profiling for fibroblasts and MSCs
[25]	Thoracic aorta; femoral artery	Dermis (healthy donor); Prostatic stromal myofibroblast cell line (ATTC, CRL-2854)	Immunophenotyping; immunomodulation (PBMC activated with PHA assay); angio-, adipo- and osteo-genesis *in vitro*	All cells expressed CD44 and FSP; similar expression of CD90 and CD105 between MSCs and myofibroblast; dermal fibroblasts completely negative; MSC unique anti-inflammatory and wound healing capacities
[26]	Bone marrow, fat, amnion, chorion, umbilical cord	Three different human skin dermis layers (dermo-hypodermal junction, intermediate reticular dermis, superficial papillary dermis)	Genome-wide transcriptome profiling	Three skin fibroblast types form clearly distinct group from five tissue-derived MSC types
[27]	Bone marrow (ATTC, PCS-500-012)	Dermis (ATTC, PCS-201-012)	Next generation RNA sequencing	Different molecular signatures between MSCs and fibroblasts; homeobox genes with important roles in embryonic development were predominantly expressed in MSCs

Reference	Source of MSCs	Source of fibroblasts	Methods	Findings
[28]	Bone marrow; endometrium and FACS-isolated cells (PDGFRβ$^+$ and CD146$^+$)	Endometrium and FACS-isolated cells (PDGFRβ$^+$ and CD146$^-$)	Immunophenotyping; cell proliferation and migration; cytokine/chemokine secretion profiling (+/-LPS)	Both types of MSCs have similar stem cell surface markers, and higher proliferation and migration potential compared to fibroblasts; bone-marrow-derived MSCs showed greater cytokine secretion after stimulation with LPS, in comparison to endometrium-derived MSCs and fibroblasts
[29]	Adipose tissue from discarded material from three different donors undergoing elective surgery	Discarded material from three different donors undergoing elective surgery	Extracellular matrix production *in vitro*; immunofluorescence for collagen type I and fibronectin; ELISA quantification of collagen I	Adipose-derived MSCs produce more fibronectin- and collagen-containing dermal matrix upon stimulation with ascorbic acid, compared to fibroblasts
[30]	Umbilical cord blood-derived MSCs (Medipost Co Ltd.)	Dermis of healthy and diabetic adults	Cell proliferation; collagen and glycosaminoglycan levels	MSC-treated group showed significantly higher collagen synthesis and glycosaminoglycan levels than fibroblast-treated group
[31]	Bone marrow (CD105 and CD271$^+$)	Male foreskin	Metabolically and hypoxia conditioned media from MSC and fibroblast migration assays	Both conditioned media have high concentrations of angiogenic factors; fibroblast-derived media attracted MSCs as efficiently as media produced by MSCs

ATTC, American Type Culture Collection; FACS, fluorescence activated cell sorting; LPS, lipopolysaccharide, PBMC, peripheral blood mononuclear cells, PHA, phytohemagglutinin; FSP, fibroblast-specific protein; PDGFRβ, platelet derived growth factor receptor β.

Table 1.
Overview of recent studies with face-to-face comparisons of various tissue-derived MSCs and fibroblasts.

2.1 Common properties: tissue remodeling and immunomodulation

In contrast to the extremely rare status of MSCs in almost all adult connective tissue (i.e., from 1 to 25 cells per 1,000,000 cells in bone marrow are MSCs [32, 33]), fibroblasts are the most abundant cell type in connective tissue [22]. Fibroblasts are the maintainers of extracellular matrix turnover, and they regulate several physiological processes. In contrast, MSCs are quiescent most of the time, but have self-renewing capacity. However, in response to certain stimuli, such as tissue injury, MSCs respond promptly, resulting in their activation and proliferation, and their differentiation into the terminal cell types that are required for regeneration following an injury [8, 33]. Both cell types can provide the stroma, in particular as collagen for tissues during injury and wound healing. However, it appears that the repair processes that result in formation of a functional tissue, such as collagen type II in cartilage injury, is a feature of MSCs, and particularly for those of the synovium [34]. Fibroblasts or other tissue-derived MSCs (e.g., bone marrow) might

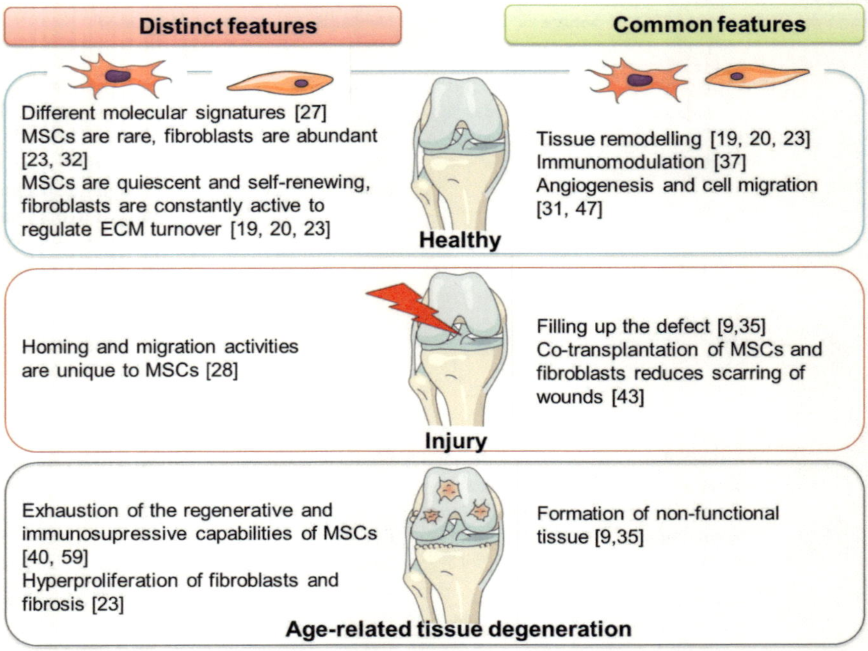

Figure 2.
Schematic representation of the distinct and common features of MSCs and fibroblasts in health and disease, with a focus on human synovial joints. ECM, extracellular matrix.

be responsible for the filling of defects in cartilage injury with only fibrous tissue; i.e., the fibrocartilage, which is a nonfunctional tissue [9, 35]. Although some early studies showed efficacy for fresh human skin allografts in the treatment of diabetic ulcers, severe burns, and other such injuries, recent studies have instead suggested that fibroblasts are more likely contaminants in such cell therapies, and thus they should be depleted so as not to impede the rejuvenation effects of stem cells [36]. There is also evidence that fibroblasts can undergo aggressive transformation in response to the tumor microenvironment, and thus contribute to disease pathophysiology, such as in cancers [22].

Immunomodulation is a fundamental characteristic of all stroma, which includes, in particular, immunosuppressive effects [37]. Jones et al. showed that stromal cells (e.g., chondrocytes, fibroblasts from synovial joints, lung, skin) can inhibit proliferation of peripheral blood mononuclear cells following polyclonal stimuli. In contrast to parenchymal cells, stromal cells showed antiproliferative functions, irrespective of their differentiation potential and/or content of progenitor cells [37].

During inflammation, proteins and lipids secreted by various cells act in a concerted fashion. Tahir et al. analyzed the formation of the most relevant inflammation mediators, including proteins and lipids, in human fibroblasts and MSCs upon inflammatory stimulation and subsequent treatment with dexamethasone [24]. They showed that fibroblasts and MSCs have similar secretion profiles for stimulation and modulation of inflammation [24].

In contrast, there are also studies that have provided evidence of greater anti-inflammatory and wound-healing features of MSCs in comparison to other stromal cells [25]. In an array of *in-vitro* tests to compare human artery-wall-derived MSCs with dermal fibroblasts and myofibroblasts, Pasanisi et al. showed some profound differences in the immunomodulatory properties between these cell types [25].

Both the dermal fibroblasts and myofibroblasts expressed very low levels of immunomodulatory and inflammation-related genes, and had lower immunosuppressive potential for proliferation of peripheral blood mononuclear cells in comparison to the femoral artery MSCs. They also suggested that the two highly sought after translational abilities, as anti-inflammatory and wound healing activities, are unique features of MSCs [25].

Although MSCs and fibroblasts share common sources for their isolation, such as adipose tissue, muscle, and skin, most recent studies have used bone marrow as the source of MSCs and skin as the source of fibroblasts. Following their plastic adherence after isolation and *in-vitro* culture expansion, fibroblasts are morphologically indistinguishable from MSCs, as they both have a spindle-shaped morphology [20]. They also both express the same positive mesenchymal markers, and both lack hematopoietic markers [19]. They also both show trilineage differentiation; i.e., adipogenesis, osteogenesis, and chondrogenesis [36]. Hence, the minimal criteria set by the International Society for Cellular Therapy to define MSCs [6] can also define fibroblasts [20]. Despite great effort, the lack of a specific marker to distinguish between MSCs and fibroblasts represents a major limit in the study of these cells [25].

2.2 Distinct properties: transcriptome profile and migration capacity

Haydont et al. recently performed a wide comparison of skin fibroblasts from three different locations in the deep dermis and hypodermis with five different tissue-derived MSCs [26]. Using genome-wide transcriptome profiling, they showed a clear 'fibroblast' molecular identity that did not segregate with the MSCs. The molecular signature that identified the fibroblasts comprised transcripts associated with hyaluronic acid, aggrecan, collagen processing, collagen fibril anchorage points, the elastic networks, and some others [26]. Similarly, using next-generation RNA sequencing, Taşkiran and Karaosmanoğlu showed that human primary bone marrow MSCs and human primary dermal fibroblasts have different molecular signatures [27]. In particular, a large group of genes that have important roles in embryonic development were highly expressed in MSCs; e.g., the homeobox genes. Aristaless-like homeobox family member ALX1 and distal-less homeobox DXL1, 5, and 6 are involved in craniofacial development, while short stature homeobox (SHOX) regulates expression of early osteogenic genes during cell differentiation. Taşkiran and Karaosmanoğlu suggested that MSCs are more appropriate for developmental and differentiation studies, compared to dermal fibroblasts [27].

Another feature that appears to be more attributed to MSCs is homing through migration. Intrinsic inflammatory characteristics have a pivotal role in stem-cell recruitment [28]. Bone marrow-derived MSCs have been demonstrated to migrate to the endometrium to contribute to the stem-cell reservoir and the regeneration of endometrial tissue [28]. Khatun et al. compared inflammation-driven migration of human bone-marrow-derived MSCs to MSCs and fibroblasts derived from the same niche (i.e., the endometrium). They showed that similar to bone-marrow-derived MSCs, endometrial MSCs showed high migration activity. However, the differentiation process toward stromal fibroblasts resulted in minimal migration [28].

3. MSCs and fibroblasts: their roles in tissue injury

A schematic representation of the interactions between MSCs and fibroblasts is shown in **Figure 3**. Following tissue injury through bone fracture, joint trauma, muscle tears, and skin wounds, for example, a well-orchestrated series

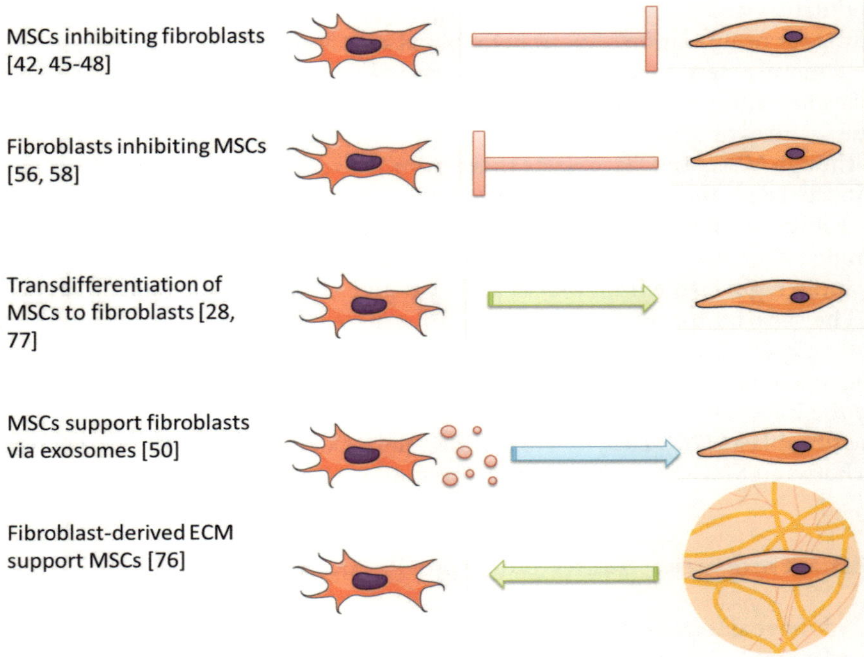

Figure 3.
Schematic representation of the interactions between MSCs and fibroblasts as observed in the in vitro studies. ECM, extracellular matrix.

of time-dependent and overlapping events takes place, including coagulation, inflammation, new tissue formation, and injury resolution. Each phase needs to be efficiently carried out to allow the further progression toward tissue regeneration.

MSCs can secrete a variety of cytokines and growth factors that have immunosuppressive and antifibrotic properties, which can have beneficial influences in the healing process [38]. The failure of tissue regeneration most commonly results in chronic inflammation and/or fibrosis, which leads to damage of the adjacent tissues and/or formation of inferior nonfunctional tissue. Some tissues have poor healing capacities if a wound extends beyond the epidermis, such as skin and cartilage, in particular. It is not entirely clear whether this is due to the absence or 'exhaustion' of the endogenous MSCs in these tissues, due to disease or age [39, 40]. Fibrosis, or scarring, is defined as accelerated accumulation of extracellular matrix factors, as predominantly collagen type I, which can prevent regeneration of tissue. This can occur in virtually any tissue as a result of trauma, inflammation, immunological rejection, chemical toxicity, or oxidative stress [38]. Following cartilage surface injury, the hyaline cartilage that is predominantly collagen type II is replaced by collagen type I, which lacks the functional properties of cartilage, such as shock absorption and reduction of friction in the joint.

The antifibrotic effects of MSCs are not entirely understood, and they are likely to overlap with the MSC anti-inflammatory and angiogenic properties [38, 41]. However, MSCs secrete several cytokines and growth factors that inhibit fibroblasts [42]. Hepatocyte growth factor released by MSCs has been shown to down-regulate the expression of transforming growth factor-β1 (TGF-β1) and collagen type I and III by fibroblasts, and on the other hand, to up-regulate expression of matrix metalloproteinases 1, 3, and 13 in fibroblasts, thereby promoting turnover of the extracellular matrix [42]. In agreement with this, Yates et al. showed that co-transplantation of MSCs and fibroblasts reduces scarring of wounds [43]. They transplanted xenogeneic MSCs and showed that these augmented fibroblast proliferation and migration, and the extracellular matrix deposition that is critical for wound closure; this co-transplantation also reduced inflammation following wounding, an effect that was greater than seen for MSCs or fibroblasts alone. These data suggested complementary roles of MSCs and fibroblasts to normalize matrix regeneration during healing, and they demonstrated that even transiently engrafted cells can have a long-term impact via matrix modulation and 'education' of other tissue cells [43].

Domaszewska-Szostek et al. recently reviewed the available data on the efficiency of cell therapies for the treatment of chronic wounds, with these therapies including fibroblasts, keratinocytes, fibroblasts and keratinocytes together, bone-marrow-derived MSCs, and adipose tissue cells [44]. They showed that the majority of reports were on fibroblasts and keratinocytes, which included cell-based products that are already on the market. Based on the knowledge at the time, Domaszewska-Szostek et al. suggested that cell therapies in the treatment of chronic wounds showed immense potential. However, much is yet to be determined from both sides, in terms of both patients and cell therapies [44].

3.1 Skin injuries

While fibroblast-based substitutes have already been used in regenerative medicine, and in particular in regeneration of skin, a recent study by Paganelli et al. suggested that adipose-tissue-derived MSCs might represent a better alternative to fibroblasts in full-thickness skin injuries [29]. They showed that *in-vitro* adipose-tissue-derived MSCs produce a collagen- and fibronectin-containing dermal matrix that is more abundant than for fibroblasts [29]. Moreover, adipose-tissue-derived MSCs also served as modulators in the regeneration of tissue that was inflamed or scarred secondary to injuries such as burns or trauma. Liu et al. investigated the effects of adipose-tissue-derived MSCs on keloidal disease, which is a particular type of scarring that is considered to arise from excessive proliferation of fibroblasts and extracellular matrix deposition [45]. They used a starvation-induced conditioned medium from adipose-tissue-derived MSCs to treat human keloid-derived fibroblasts, and evaluated the fibroblast *in-vitro* proliferation, migration, and apoptosis. These human keloid-derived fibroblasts showed inhibited proliferation and collagen synthesis. They also used a keloid xenograft implantation animal model to assess the paracrine effects of conditioned medium from adipose-tissue-derived MSCs *in vivo*. They noted reduced inflammation and fibrosis in an *in-vivo* keloid model, which was seen as keloid shrinkage and reduced inflammatory cell accumulation, blood vessel density, and collagen deposition [45].

Han et al. took things a step further, and included a photobiomodulation pretreatment of adipose-derived MSCs before collection of their conditioned medium. Photobiomodulation is a laser treatment that uses low power and energy, but has been shown to induce positive photobiological processes in cells, such as regulation of cell secretion, and promotion of cell proliferation, differentiation, and migration, with enhanced immunological functions, and therefore, accelerated tissue repair [46]. However, when they cultured hypertrophic scar and keloid fibroblasts in conditioned medium from adipose MSCs pretreated with photobiomodulation therapy for 12, 24, and 48 h, there was inhibition of proliferation of these fibroblasts, and down-regulation of their profibrotic growth factors and collagen synthesis. They also suggested that the mechanism for this inhibition was related to down-regulation of TGF-β1 and Notch-1 expression [46].

In addition to adipose-tissue-derived MSCs, bone-marrow-derived MSC have shown benefits for keloids and hypertrophic scars. Fang et al. showed that bone-marrow-derived MSCs use a paracrine signaling mechanism to attenuate the fibroblast proliferative and profibrotic phenotypes derived from hypertrophic scars and keloids, and to inhibit extracellular matrix synthesis [47]. Using conditioned medium from bone-marrow MSCs, they showed significant inhibition of proliferation and migration of the fibroblasts from hypertrophic scars and keloids, in comparison with the use of conditioned medium from normal skin fibroblasts. Furthermore, they also reported that for conditioned medium from bone-marrow-derived MSCs, for both of these types of fibroblasts, there was decreased expression of profibrotic genes, including those for connective tissue growth factor, plasminogen activator inhibitor-1, TGF-β1, and TGF-β2, and increased expression of antifibrotic genes, including those for TGF-β3 and decorin. Moreover, they reported decreased expression of collagen I and fibronectin and low levels of hydroxyproline in the cell culture supernatant, which suggested that the conditioned medium from bone MSCs suppressed the synthesis of extracellular matrix in these fibroblasts [47].

Similar data were reported by Sato et al. for amnion-derived MSCs. Following harvesting of keloid, mature and normal fibroblasts, and their stimulation with TGF-β, they showed that conditioned medium obtained from the amnion-derived MSCs prevented proliferation and activation of the keloid fibroblasts [48].

Tooi et al. used a similar study design; however, they used conditioned medium from human placenta-derived MSCs to harvest exosomes, and examined their effects on normal adult dermal fibroblasts *in vitro* [49]. Exosomes contain nucleic acids, proteins, and lipids, and function as an intercellular communication vehicle for mediation of the paracrine effects of MSCs [49]. They reported positive effects of this treatment, and in particular, significant up-regulation of stemness-related genes, such as octamer-binding transcription factor 4 (Oct4) and NANOG homebox gene, and differentiation competence of fibroblasts to adipocytes and osteoblasts [49].

Hu et al. investigated the roles of exosomes derived from adipose MSCs in cutaneous wound healing [50]. *In vitro*, they showed that these exosomes can be taken up and internalized by fibroblasts, to stimulate cell migration and proliferation, and collagen synthesis, in a dose-dependent manner. *In vivo*, they demonstrated that these exosomes can be recruited to soft tissue wound areas in a mouse skin incision model, and that they significantly accelerated cutaneous wound healing. Following systemic administration of exosomes, they reported increased collagen I and III production in the early stage of wound healing, and inhibited collagen expression in the late stage, which might be favorable to reduce scar formation. Based on these results, they suggested that exomes can be used to facilitate cutaneous wound healing via optimizing the characteristics of fibroblasts [50].

Li et al. explored the paracrine effects of conditioned medium from umbilical-cord-derived MSCs on dermal fibroblasts [51]. They showed that this treatment increased the proliferation and migration of fibroblasts. Moreover, they also reported on their transition into a phenotype with a low myofibroblast formation capacity, a decreased ratio of TGF-β1/3, and an increased ratio of matrix metalloproteinase/ tissue inhibitor of metalloproteinases. They also performed *in-vivo* wound healing assays. Full thickness skin excisional wounds treated with conditioned medium from umbilical-cord-derived MSCs showed accelerated healing, with fewer scars seen.

Pan et al. investigated the effects of conditioned medium derived from human amniotic MSCs on hydrogen-peroxide-induced senescence of human dermal fibroblasts. They showed that the conditioned medium derived from these cells significantly decreased senescence-associated β-galactosidase activity, and promoted proliferation of senescent human dermal fibroblasts [52]. Interestingly, they also showed the same effect using conditioned medium from human amniotic epithelial cells. These cells were isolated from the same amniotic tissue, and characterized by their similar immunophenotype to the MSCs, except for stage-specific embryonic antigen-4 as specific to MSCs, and their cobblestone-like morphology, in contrast to the MSC fibroblast morphology [52].

Gabrielyan et al. directly compared metabolically conditioned medium and hypoxia-conditioned medium derived from bone-marrow MSCs and skin fibroblasts, and evaluated their attraction of bone-marrow MSCs in two-dimensional migration assays [31]. They reported that the conditioned media from both types of cells had high concentrations of the angiogenic factors that are important for angiogenesis and cell migration. Having shown that both of the conditioned media produced by human skin fibroblasts attracted MSCs as efficiently as conditioned medium produced by human bone-marrow MSCs, these authors favored fibroblasts-derived metabolic conditioning as providing easier, cheaper, and faster access to chemoattractive agents [31].

3.2 Diabetic wounds

There are also several studies that have suggested superior effects of MSCs compared to fibroblasts for the stimulation of diabetic wound healing [30, 53]. Jung et al. compared the treatment effects of human umbilical-cord-blood-derived MSCs with those of fibroblasts on diabetic wound healing *in vitro* [30]. Using co-culture of diabetic fibroblasts with either healthy fibroblasts or umbilical-cord-blood-derived MSCs over 3 days, they measured cell proliferation and collagen synthesis and glycosaminoglycan levels, which are the major contributing factors to wound healing. The group treated with the umbilical-cord-blood-derived MSCs showed significantly greater collagen synthesis and glycosaminoglycan levels than the fibroblast-treated group [30]. Saheli et al. also focused on the interplay between MSCs and fibroblasts in diabetic wound healing, in both *in-vivo* and *in-vitro* diabetic models [53]. *In vivo*, in the group of diabetic wounds treated with MSC-derived conditioned medium, they demonstrated significantly greater wound closure, less pronounced inflammatory responses in the granulation tissue, better tissue remodeling, and more vascularization, compared with the nontreated diabetic wounds [53]. *In vitro*, they cultured human dermal fibroblasts in a high-glucose medium. When these fibroblasts were incubated in the presence of MSC-derived conditioned medium, they showed up-regulation of the genes encoding epidermal growth factor and basic fibroblast growth factor (bFGF), in addition to significantly greater cell viability/ proliferation, and migration. Based on these findings, they suggested that MSC-derived conditioned medium improves the activity of the fibroblasts in the diabetic microenvironment, and thus might promote wound repair and skin regeneration [53].

3.3 Ligament injuries

Similar to cartilage, ligaments have poor healing capacity due to hypocellularity and lack of cellular components for self-regeneration. Li et al. investigated differentiation of human amnion-derived MSCs into human anterior cruciate ligament fibroblasts *in vitro* using a Transwell co-culture system and induction with bFGF and TGF-β1 [54]. Following an array of gene and protein expression for ligament-specific molecules, they suggested Transwell co-cultures as an optimal system for differentiation of amnion-derived MSCs into ligament fibroblasts [54].

3.4 Periodontal disease and jaw injuries

Osteoradionecrosis of the jaw is a severe chronic adverse effect of ionizing radiation therapy to the head and neck region. It is manifested as soft tissue fibrosis, chronic inflammation of the bone, and osteonecrosis of the maxillofacial region, with histopathological formation phases that are very similar to those of chronic wounds [55]. Zhuang and Zou reported inhibitory effects of irradiation-activated-gingival fibroblasts on osteogenic differentiation of human bone-derived MSCs [56]. They showed that exosome-mediated delivery of miR-23a from irradiation-activated fibroblasts inhibited osteogenesis of bone MSCs via directly targeting C-X-C motif chemokine ligand 12 (CXCL12) [56]. Under this pathological condition, rather than working hand in hand, fibroblasts and MSCs appeared to be on opposing sides of the tissue healing process.

A similar situation has been reported for periodontal diseases. These encompass a wide variety of chronic inflammatory conditions in the gingiva (i.e., soft tissue surrounding the teeth) and the periodontal connective tissues, such as the bone and ligaments [57]. Periodontal disease begins with gingivitis, as localized inflammation of the gingiva that is initiated by bacteria in the dental plaque. If untreated, gingivitis can progress to loss of the gingiva, bone and ligaments, which creates the deep periodontal 'pockets' that are a hallmark of this disease, and which can eventually lead to tooth loss [57]. Periodontal ligaments have MSCs that can form fibroblasts, cementoblasts, and osteoblasts, and can thus be used for periodontal regenerative therapy. However, the fate of their differentiation is under the control of the periodontal cells, either via direct contact or via secretion of humoral factors. Kaneda-Ikeda et al. clarified the regulatory mechanism for MSC differentiation by humoral factors from gingival fibroblasts [58]. They indirectly co-cultured human ilium-derived MSCs with human gingival fibroblasts under osteogenic or growth conditions. Interestingly, they reported that humoral factors released by gingival fibroblasts suppressed osteogenesis of MSCs. This effect was regulated by miRNAs and undifferentiated MSC markers [58].

4. MSCs and fibroblasts: their roles in age-related tissue degeneration

With aging, and in particular with degenerative disorders of the musculoskeletal system such as osteoarthritis and osteoporosis, MSCs appear to be 'exhausted', with a lack of regenerative potential [33, 40, 59], or their regenerative potential is diverted from functional to production of nonfunctional cell types, such as adipocytes and fibroblasts [60, 61]. Fibroblasts, on the other hand undergo hyperproliferation resulting in age-related fibrosis of many tissues and organs, in particularly skin, lung, kidney, liver and heart [23].

4.1 Intravertebral disc degeneration

Degeneration of the intervertebral discs is strongly implicated as a cause of lower back pain, which has been shown to affect up to 85% of people at some point during their lives [62]. Although it is most commonly manifested in adulthood and its progression is closely linked to aging, changes in the cellular microenvironment of the discs can begin as early as a few years after birth [62]. Inflammation has been correlated with degenerative disc disease, but its role in discogenic pain and hernia regression remains controversial. Inflammatory responses might be involved in the onset of the disease, although it is also crucial for maintenance of tissue homeostasis [63].

Clinical studies that have used autologous or allogeneic MSCs to treat patients with back pain have reported some encouraging results [64]. There is also evidence that fibroblasts injected into the degenerated discs remain viable, and thus might represent an effective therapy for prevention or for delay of degenerative diseases of the discs. However these data were obtained in animal models only [65].

Shi et al. showed that transplantation of human dermal fibroblasts into degenerating intervertebral discs of rabbits can significantly increase the markers of disc regeneration (e.g., disc height, collagen type I and II gene expression, proteoglycan content). In comparison to transplantation of rabbit dermal fibroblasts, these results showed similar regenerative trends, but these trends did not reach significant difference. This study also showed that the human cells transplanted into rabbit discs did not induce immune response in the rabbit cells [66].

4.2 Bone degeneration

In addition to disc degeneration, most elderly people develop bone loss with age [54]. The most common clinical manifestation of bone loss is osteoporosis associated with an increased risk of fractures, which can also lead to death. In 2017, new fragility fractures in the EU6 were estimated at 2.7 million, with an associated annual cost of €37.5 billion and a loss of 1.0 million quality-adjusted life years [67]. As osteoblasts have a central role in the process of bone formation, the direct reprogramming of fibroblasts into osteoblasts might be a new way to treat bone fractures in elderly individuals. Chang et al. recently reviewed a large body of literature and proposed several clinical applications of a direct conversion method for generating osteoblasts in patients [68]. Successful direct conversion of fibroblasts into osteoblasts was reported previously in 2015, using defined transcription factors, such as Osterix, runt-related transcription factor 2 (Runx2), Oct3/4, and L-myc [69]. Despite this, Chang et al. concluded that more work is needed to determine the best way to directly reprogram somatic cells into osteoblasts for optimal clinical use. They also suggested that in addition to successful fibroblast-to-osteoblast conversion, future studies will need to consider the optimal cellular microenvironment to promote osteoblast survival and bone formation in patients [68]. The microenvironment is a common component and factor with immense importance for efficacy of cell therapies of any kind [70].

5. MSCs and fibroblasts: their roles in immunological disorders

5.1 Rheumatoid arthritis

Under normal conditions, the joint membrane, i.e. synovium represent the site of the two closely related cell types: i.e., fibroblast-like synoviocytes and synovial MSCs. These can work hand in hand as immunomodulatory cells to control the magnitude of immune responses. Rheumatoid arthritis is a chronic autoimmune disease that manifests as polyarthritis with joint destruction [71]. The main pathological characteristic of this rheumatic disease is increased proliferation of fibroblasts and accumulation of inflammatory cells, which results in the formation of the 'pannus'. Interestingly, based on the evidence from animal models, Matsuo et al. suggested that resident fibroblasts account for the pathology of rheumatoid arthritis, and not bone-marrow-derived and circulating cells [71]. In addition, genetic lineage tracing studies have suggested that fibroblasts in rheumatoid arthritis originate from local proliferation of resident fibroblasts, differentiation of pericytes and MSCs, and transition of endothelial cells [71]. The main targets in this disease are thus inflammatory cytokines and leukocytes. As MSCs are immunosuppressive, they have great potential in therapies for this inflammatory disease [72]. However, it appears that the swamping of the microenvironment in rheumatoid arthritis with inflammatory cells and cytokines causes loss of efficacy in the responses of the endogenous joint-resident MSCs to the exaggerated immune response. In addition, synovial fibroblasts are likely to derive from synovial-membrane-derived MSCs, which can also to give rise to fibroblast-like synoviocytes, as key players in perpetuation of joint inflammation and destruction in rheumatoid arthritis [73].

5.2 Systemic sclerosis

Systemic sclerosis is a rare autoimmune rheumatic disease that is characterized by excessive production and accumulation of collagen in different tissues. The physiopathology of systemic sclerosis has still not been completely elucidated, although roles for fibroblasts, endothelial cells, immune cells, and oxidative stress have been demonstrated [74]. Several studies have established the beneficial effects of administration of MSCs from various tissue sources in different preclinical models that are characterized by local or systemic fibrosis. Clinical studies are, however, still falling behind. On the other hand, MSCs from patients with systemic sclerosis have been shown to constitutively express factors that stimulate fibrotic and angiogenic processes. This might indicate that MSCs are altered by the environment secondary to the onset of the disease, or that they might participate in the physiopathology of the disease [75]. Hence, the rationale for using allogenic MSCs in systemic sclerosis (as well as in other autoimmune diseases) is based on the possibility that autologous MSCs will be altered in these diseases [74].

6. MSCs and fibroblasts: how to boost their complementary tissue regeneration

6.1 In-vitro *approaches*

As MSCs represent rare cell populations *in vivo*, their *in-vitro* expansion is an often-unavoidable step in the preparation for these cell therapies. Currently, MSC expansion is most commonly achieved via cultivation on tissue culture plastics with the addition of 10% fetal bovine serum. Van et al. investigated the feasibility of human fibroblast-derived extracellular matrix as an alternative for *in-vitro* cell expansion [76]. Such fibroblast-derived extracellular matrix was obtained from decellularized extracellular matrix derived from *in-vitro*-cultured human lung fibroblasts. Using umbilical-cord-blood-derived MSCs, they directly compared cell cultivation on tissue culture plastics, fibronectin-coated tissue culture plastics, and human fibroblast-derived extracellular matrix. They showed that the last of these, the human fibroblast-derived extracellular matrix, improved cell proliferation, migration, and osteogenesis, as well as the expression of stemness and engraftment-related markers of MSCs. Furthermore, they showed superior *in-vivo* effects of MSCs pre-conditioned on human fibroblast-derived matrix in an emphysema animal model (i.e., a lung disease). Based on this, they suggested that human fibroblast-derived matrix represents a naturally derived biomimetic microenvironment with potential for practical applications in regenerative medicine [76].

Adipose-derived MSCs represent the preferable autologous source of MSCs in regenerative medicine in general, due to their indispensability in adults. Sivan et al. standardized their *in-vitro* culture conditions for differentiation of adipose-derived MSCs into dermal-like fibroblasts, which can synthesize extracellular matrix proteins [77]. Given that adipose-derived MSCs are multipotent in nature and might develop into undesirable tissues upon transplantation, the diverting of these MSCs to a more committed, fibroblast lineage appears like a better option in skin tissue engineering. To promote commitment of these MSCs into fibroblasts, they used a special biomimetic matrix composite that was pre-coated with fibrinogen, fibronectin, gelatin, hyaluronic acid, and human platelet growth factors. When MSCs were cultured on this composite with the presence of differentiation medium supplemented with fibroblast-conditioned medium and growth factors, they showed up-regulation of fibroblast-specific protein-1 and a panel of extracellular matrix molecules that were specific to the dermis, such as fibrillin-1, collagen I, collagen IV, and elastin. As fibroblasts derived from adipose MSCs can synthesize elastin, this is an added advantage for successful skin tissue engineering, compared to fibroblasts from skin biopsies [77].

To boost the combined tissue-healing effects of MSCs and fibroblasts, several tissue engineering approaches are being investigated. To enhance resistance to oxidative stress and the paracrine potential of MSCs, Costa et al. formulated MSC spheroids encapsulated in alginate microbeads [78]. This three-dimensional formulation showed increased angiogenic and chemotactic potential relative to encapsulated single cells. As the encapsulated MSCs promoted formation of tube-like structures and migration of fibroblasts into the wounded area, these authors suggested that such a model setting can be used for wound repair and regeneration processes [78].

As oxygen represents an important factor in tissue healing, hyperbaric oxygen therapy is an effective adjunct treatment for ischemic disorders, such as chronic wounds. Engel et al. showed beneficial effects of hyperbaric oxygen therapy on mono-cultures and co-cultures of human adipose-derived MSCs and fibroblasts [79]. The results of this study suggested that hyperbaric oxygen therapy leads to immunomodulatory and proangiogenetic effects in a wound-like environment, where adipose-derived MSCs and fibroblasts collaborated toward efficient wound healing [79].

In addition to cell therapies where formulation for clinical use still represents immense challenges, great hope has also been put into the cell-free formulations for use in regenerative medicine. Several studies have explored the effects of conditioned media from various tissue-derived MSCs on fibroblasts (as described in 3.1). Conditioned medium is a cell-free formulation, and it basically defines the adult stem-cell secretome.The majority of studies that used conditioned medium to enhance fibroblast properties, harvested the medium from two-dimensional cultures of MSCs from various tissue sources. Using a polystyrene scaffold, Kim et al. created a three-dimensional culture of perivascular cells, which represented a more physiologically appropriate system to harvest conditioned medium [80]. They used this medium to investigate the effects on the migration and proliferation of human keratinocytes and fibroblasts. The migration of both of these types of cells, and also the proliferation of keratinocytes, were significantly greater with the conditioned medium from this three-dimensional culture system. They also reported greater expression of type I collagen, specific expression of some other factors (e.g., thioredoxin), and more small particles such as CD63-positive extracellular vesicles, which were shown to stimulate keratinocyte migration. Based on these data, the three-dimensional cultures have the potential to be considered as future wound-healing remedies.

An *in-vivo* alternative to conditioned medium produced by *in-vitro* cultured MSCs was tested by Cerny et al. [81]. They used wound fluid samples from fingertip injuries and split skin donor sites under occlusive dressings, to evaluate the effects of paracrine factors in the wound fluid (secretome) on migration and proliferation of MSCs and fibroblasts. Under these conditions, MSCs showed significant increases in both migration and proliferation, while fibroblasts showed a significant increase in migration only. Hence, the paracrine factors in the wound fluid can modulate the wound-healing process, and can reduce scar-tissue formation [81].

6.2 In-vivo *approaches*

When it comes to *in-vivo* approaches to stimulate endogenous MSCs and fibroblasts, platelet-rich plasma has been widely studied and is used in clinical practice. Platelet-rich plasma contains higher concentrations of platelets than whole blood, as typically three-fold to five-fold higher compared with normal plasma (normal: 150,000 to 300,000 platelets per microliter) [82]. This platelet concentrate has been shown to have anti-inflammatory effects through growth factors, such as TGF-β and insulin-like growth factor 1, and also stimulatory effects on MSCs and fibroblasts [82].

Stessuk et al. evaluated the combined effects of platelet-rich plasma and conditioned medium from adipose-derived MSCs on fibroblasts and keratinocytes *in vitro*. They showed significant proliferation of both cell types, and also significant migration of fibroblasts treated with both components, which suggested the potential of this combination for healing and re-epithelialization of chronic wounds *in vivo* [83].

The major issue of unpredictable and difficult-to-replicate *in-vivo* effects of MSC therapies is most probably the microenvironment that these cell injections are delivered into. In healthy tissues, stem cells reside within a complex microenvironment that comprises cellular, structural, and signaling cues that collectively maintain stemness and modulate tissue homeostasis [70]. Following tissue injury, substantial changes are made to this unique cell environment, which will influence the regulation of stem-cell differentiation, trophic signaling, and tissue healing. Bogdanowicz and Lu reviewed recent studies on how microenvironmental cues modulate MSC responses following connective tissue injury, and how this microenvironment can be programmed for stem-cell-guided tissue regeneration [70]. Based on their revised data, these authors suggested that the cell microenvironment should be conducive to stem-cell lineage commitment, biomimetic tissue regeneration, and ultimately, restoration of physiological functions. In this light, specific attention should be directed to methods for standardization of experimental conditions both *in vitro* and *in vivo*, and in particular to optimization of cell seeding densities and cell sources [70].

To mimic the optimal microenvironment for MSCs, several novel technological approaches are being developed. Combining human fibroblast-derived matrix and the biocompatible polymer hydrogel (i.e., polyvinyl alcohol), Ha et al. demonstrated cytocompatibility with human MSCs [84]. Moreover, this advanced wound healing therapy was shown to be efficient in full-thickness wound repair in a preclinical model [84].

6.3 Converting fibroblasts to MSCs

When it comes to vascular damage, vascular-wall-derived MSCs might be particularly well suited for resolution of such injuries. Recently, Steens et al. developed a method for direct conversion of human skin fibroblasts into vascular MSCs. They directed cell-fate conversion through induction of ectopic expression of the highly vascular MSC-specific *HOX* genes, including HOXB7, HOXC6, and HOXC8, while bypassing pluripotency. The converted MSCs showed classical multipotent MSC characteristics *in vitro* (i.e., multipotency, clonogenicity), and were selectively associated with vascular structures *in vivo*. With respect to their therapeutic potential, these cells suppressed lymphocyte proliferation *in vitro*, while in a mouse model of radiation-induced pneumopathy *in vivo*, they protected the mice against vascular damage, as also for *ex-vivo* cultured human lung tissue [85]. These data suggested an efficient strategy for treatment of vascular diseases, such as hypertension, ischemic diseases, vascular lesions, and others.

In addition to genetic manipulation to convert fibroblasts to MSCs, there is also a chemical method available to convert primary human dermal fibroblasts into multipotent, induced MSC-like cells. Using a defined cocktail of small molecules and growth factors, (six chemical inhibitors, plus TGF-β, bFGF, and leukemia inhibitory factor), Lai et al. converted human fibroblasts into inducible MSCs in a monolayer culture over 6 days, with 38% conversion rate [86]. The inducible MSCs behaved like primary bone-marrow-derived MSCs in terms of their multipotency, clonogenicity, molecular signatures, and surface marker expression profile. Moreover, these MSCs were as effectively as bone-marrow-derived MSCs in their significant protection against fatality with endotoxin-induced acute lung injury in a mouse model. Based on these data, the authors suggested that this chemical conversion of fibroblasts to MSCs is superior to the genetic approach, as this latter might have the risk of insertional mutagenesis [86].

7. Conclusions

The relative failure of decades-long endeavors to establish a clear definition for both MSCs and fibroblasts appears to be a result of the complementary and overlapping roles these cells have in cell homeostasis and tissue development and injury. Indeed, due to the similarities in their morphologies, immunophenotypes, and connective tissue stroma formation, MSCs and fibroblasts are indistinguishable in most *in-vitro* settings. However, *in-vivo* studies, and in particular recent studies using modern analytics such as next-generation sequencing, have indicated that a line can be drawn to distinguish between MSCs and fibroblasts. On the other hand, several studies have demonstrated that it is the cellular therapies that combine both of these cell types that represent the optimal approach for future development of tissue-regenerating strategies.

Acknowledgements

Janja Zupan was funded by UK Arthritis Research (2016–2018) and is currently part of the P3-0298 Research Programme "Genes, hormones and personality changes in metabolic disorders", and is Leader of the J3-1749 Research Project "Mesenchymal stem cells-the keepers of tissue endogenous regenerative capacity facing up to aging of the musculoskeletal system", both, funded by the Slovenian Research Agency. The author would like to thank Chris Berrie for scientific English editing of the manuscript.

Conflicts of interest

The author declares that there are no conflicts of interest.

Nomenclature

bFGF	basic fibroblast growth factor
CXCL12	C-X-C motif chemokine ligand 12
MSCs	mesenchymal stem/stromal cells
OCT-4	octamer-binding transcription factor 4
SHOX	short stature homeobox
TGF-β1	transforming growth factor β1

Author details

Janja Zupan
Faculty of Pharmacy, Department of Clinical Biochemistry, University of Ljubljana, Ljubljana, Slovenia

*Address all correspondence to: janja.zupan@ffa.uni-lj.si

References

[1] Bianco P, Cao X, Frenette PS, Mao JJ, Robey PG, Simmons PJ, et al. The meaning, the sense and the significance: translating the science of mesenchymal stem cells into medicine. Nat Med 2013;19(1):35-42. https://www.nature.com/articles/nm.3028.pdf

[2] Friedenstein AJ, Chailakhjan RK, Lalykina KS. The development of fibroblast colonies in monolayer cultures of guinea pig bone marrow and spleen cells. Cell Prolif 1970;3(4):393-403.

[3] Pittenger M, Mackay A, Beck S, Jaiswal R, Douglas R, Mosca J, et al. Multilineage potential of adult human mesenchymal stem cells. Science 1999;284(5411):143-7. http://dx.doi.org/10.1126/science.284.5411.143

[4] Caplan AI. Mesenchymal stem cells. J Orthop Res 1991;9(5):641-50. http://doi.wiley.com/10.1002/jor.1100090504

[5] Caplan AI. Mesenchymal stem cells: time to change the Name! Stem Cells Transl Med 2017;6(6):1445-51. http://www.ncbi.nlm.nih.gov/pubmed/284522046.

[6] Dominici M, Le Blanc K, Mueller I, Slaper-Cortenbach I, Marini F, Krause D, et al. Minimal criteria for defining multipotent mesenchymal stromal cells. The International Society for Cellular Therapy position statement. Cytotherapy2006;8(4):315-7. http://www.ncbi.nlm.nih.gov/pubmed/16923606

[7] Viswanathan S, Shi Y, Galipeau J, Krampera M, Leblanc K. Mesenchymal stem versus stromal cells : International Society for Cell & Gene Therapy (ISCT Ò) Mesenchymal Stromal Cell committee. Cytotherapy 2019;21(10):1019-24. https://doi.org/10.1016/j.jcyt.2019.08.002

[8] Chan CKF, Gulati GS, Sinha R, Tompkins JV, Lopez M, Carter AC, et al. Identification of the human skeletal stem cell. Cell 2018;175(1):43-56.e21. http://www.ncbi.nlm.nih.gov/pubmed/30241615

[9] Murphy MP, Koepke LS, Lopez MT, Tong X, Ambrosi TH, Gulati GS, et al. Articular cartilage regeneration by activated skeletal stem cells. Nat Med 2020;26(10):1583-92. https://www.nature.com/articles/s41591-020-1013-2

[10] Crisan M, Yap S, Casteilla L, Chen CW, Corselli M, Park TS, et al. A perivascular origin for mesenchymal stem cells in multiple human organs. Cell Stem Cell 2008;3(3):301-13. https://www.sciencedirect.com/science/article/pii/S1934590908003378?via%3Dihub

[11] Guimarães-Camboa N, Cattaneo P, Sun Y, Moore-Morris T, Gu Y, Dalton ND, et al. Pericytes of multiple organs do not behave as mesenchymal stem cells in vivo. Cell Stem Cell 2017;20(3):345-359.e5. https://pubmed.ncbi.nlm.nih.gov/28111199/

[12] Pizzute T, Lynch K, Pei M. Impact of tissue-specific stem cells on lineage-specific differentiation: a focus on the musculoskeletal system. Stem Cell Rev Reports 2015;11(1):119-32. /pmc/articles/PMC4326629/

[13] Sacchetti B, Funari A, Remoli C, Giannicola G, Kogler G, Liedtke S, et al. No identical "mesenchymal stem cells" at different times and sites: human committed progenitors of distinct origin and differentiation potential are incorporated as adventitial cells in microvessels. Stem Cell Reports 2016;6(6):897-913. https://www.sciencedirect.com/science/article/pii/S2213671116300662?via%3Dihub

[14] Burja B, Barlič A, Erman A, Mrak-Poljšak K, Tomšič M,

Sodin-Semrl S, et al. Human mesenchymal stromal cells from different tissues exhibit unique responses to different inflammatory stimuli. Curr Res Transl Med 2020;68(4):217-24. https://www.sciencedirect.com/science/article/pii/S2452318620300398

[15] Deans RJ, Gunter KC, Dominici M, Forte M. Part 5: Unproven cell therapies and the commercialization of cell-based products. Cytotherapy 2016;18(1): 138-42. http://dx.doi.org/10.1016/j.jcyt.2015.11.001

[16] Sipp D, Robey PG, Turner L. Clear up this stem-cell mess. Nature 2018;561(7724):455-7. https://www.nature.com/articles/d41586-018-06756-9

[17] Molenaar JC. From the library of the Netherlands Journal of Medicine. Rudolf Virchow: Die Cellularpathologie in ihrer Begründung auf physiologische und pathologische Gewebelehre; 1858. Ned Tijdschr Geneeskd 2003;147(45): 2236-44. https://pubmed.ncbi.nlm.nih.gov/14640063/

[18] Haniffa MA, Collin MP, Buckley CD, Dazzi F. Mesenchymal stem cells: the fibroblasts' new clothes? Haematologica 2009;94(2):258-63.

[19] Denu RA, Nemcek S, Bloom DD, Goodrich AD, Kim J, Mosher DF, et al. Fibroblasts and Mesenchymal Stromal/Stem Cells Are Phenotypically Indistinguishable. Acta Haematol 2016;136(2):85-97. https://pubmed.ncbi.nlm.nih.gov/27188909/

[20] Soundararajan M, Kannan S. Fibroblasts and mesenchymal stem cells: two sides of the same coin? J Cell Physiol 2018;233(12):9099-109.

[21] Frank-Bertoncelj M, Trenkmann M, Klein K, Karouzakis E, Rehrauer H, Bratus A, et al. Epigenetically-driven anatomical diversity of synovial fibroblasts guides joint-specific fibroblast functions. Nat Commun 2017;8(1):1-14. www.nature.com/naturecommunications

[22] Aghakhani S, Zerrouk N, Niarakis A. Metabolic reprogramming of fibroblasts as therapeutic target in rheumatoid arthritis and cancer: deciphering key mechanisms using computational systems biology approaches. Cancers (Basel) 2020;13(1):35. https://www.mdpi.com/2072-6694/13/1/35

[23] Ichim TE, O'Heeron P, Kesari S. Fibroblasts as a practical alternative to mesenchymal stem cells. J Transl Med 2018;16(1):1-9. https://doi.org/10.1186/s12967-018-1536-1

[24] Tahir A, Bileck A, Muqaku B, Niederstaetter L, Kreutz D, Mayer RL, et al. Combined proteome and eicosanoid profiling approach for revealing implications of human fibroblasts in chronic inflammation. Anal Chem 2017;89(3):1945-54. https://pubmed.ncbi.nlm.nih.gov/28208246/

[25] Pasanisi E, Ciavarella C, Valente S, Ricci F, Pasquinelli G. Differentiation and plasticity of human vascular wall mesenchymal stem cells, dermal fibroblasts and myofibroblasts: a critical comparison including ultrastructural evaluation of osteogenic potential. Ultrastruct Pathol 2019;43(6):261-72. https://pubmed.ncbi.nlm.nih.gov/31589079/

[26] Haydont V, Neiveyans V, Perez P, Busson É, Lataillade JJ, Asselineau D, et al. Fibroblasts from the human skin dermo-hypodermal junction are distinct from dermal papillary and reticular fibroblasts and from mesenchymal stem cells and exhibit a specific molecular Profile Related to Extracellular Matrix Organization and modeling. Cells 2020;9(2):368. https://pubmed.ncbi.nlm.nih.gov/32033496/

[27] Taşkiran EZ, Karaosmanoğlu B. Transcriptome analysis reveals differentially expressed genes between human primary bone marrow mesenchymal stem cells and human primary dermal fibroblasts. Turkish J Biol 2019;43(1):21-7. /pmc/articles/PMC6426640/

[28] Khatun M, Sorjamaa A, Kangasniemi M, Sutinen M, Salo T, Liakka A, et al. Niche matters: the comparison between bone marrow stem cells and endometrial stem cells and stromal fibroblasts reveal distinct migration and cytokine profiles in response to inflammatory stimulus. PLoS One 2017;12(4):e0175986. https://pubmed.ncbi.nlm.nih.gov/28419140/

[29] Paganelli A, Benassi L, Rossi E, Magnoni C. Extracellular matrix deposition by adipose-derived stem cells and fibroblasts: a comparative study. Arch Dermatol Res 2020;312(4):295-9. https://doi.org/10.1007/s00403-019-01997-8

[30] Jung JA, Yoon YD, Lee HW, Kang SR, Han SK. Comparison of human umbilical cord blood-derived mesenchymal stem cells with healthy fibroblasts on wound-healing activity of diabetic fibroblasts. Int Wound J [Internet]. 2018 Feb 1 [cited 2021 Jun 3];15(1):133-9. Available from: https://pubmed.ncbi.nlm.nih.gov/29115054/

[31] Gabrielyan A, Neumann E, Gelinsky M, Rösen-Wolff A. Metabolically conditioned media derived from bone marrow stromal cells or human skin fibroblasts act as effective chemoattractants for mesenchymal stem cells. Stem Cell Res Ther 2017;8(1):212. https://pubmed.ncbi.nlm.nih.gov/28969687/

[32] Worthley DL, Churchill M, Compton JT, Tailor Y, Rao M, Si Y, et al. Gremlin 1 identifies a skeletal stem cell with bone, cartilage, and reticular stromal potential. Cell 2015;160(1-2):269-84. http://dx.doi.org/10.1016/j.cell.2014.11.042

[33] Čamernik K, Barlič A, Drobnič M, Marc J, Jeras M, Zupan J. Mesenchymal stem cells in the musculoskeletal system: from animal models to human tissue regeneration? Stem Cell Rev Reports 2018;14(3):346-69. https://doi.org/10.1007/s12015-018-9800-6

[34] Roelofs AJ, Zupan J, Riemen AHK, Kania K, Ansboro S, White N, et al. Joint morphogenetic cells in the adult mammalian synovium. Nat Commun 2017;8:15040. https://www.nature.com/articles/ncomms15040.pdf

[35] Mithoefer K, Mcadams T, Williams RJ, Kreuz PC, Mandelbaum BR. Clinical efficacy of the microfracture technique for articular cartilage repair in the knee: an evidence-based systematic analysis. Am J Sports Med 2009;37(10):2053-63. https://pubmed.ncbi.nlm.nih.gov/19251676/

[36] Brohem CA, De Carvalho CM, Radoski CL, Santi FC, Baptista MC, Swinka BB, et al. Comparison between fibroblasts and mesenchymal stem cells derived from dermal and adipose tissue. Int J Cosmet Sci 2013;35(5):448-57.

[37] Jones S, Horwood N, Cope A, Dazzi F. The antiproliferative effect of mesenchymal stem cells is a fundamental property shared by all stromal cells. J Immunol 2007;179(5):2824-31. http://www.jimmunol.org/content/179/5/2824

[38] Spees JL, Lee RH, Gregory CA. Mechanisms of mesenchymal stem/stromal cell function. Stem Cell Res Ther 2016;7(1):125. https://stemcellres.biomedcentral.com/articles/10.1186/s13287-016-0363-7

[39] Čamernik K, Mihelič A, Mihalič R, Marolt Presen D, Janež A, Trebše R, et al. Increased exhaustion of the subchondral bone-derived

mesenchymal stem/ stromal cells in primary versus dysplastic osteoarthritis. Stem Cell Rev Reports 2020;16(4): 742-54. https://doi.org/10.1007/s12015-020-09964-x

[40] Partridge L, Deelen J, Slagboom PE. Facing up to the global challenges of ageing. Nature 2018;561(7721):45-56. http://www.nature.com/articles/s41586-018-0457-8

[41] Ayala-Cuellar AP, Kang JH, Jeung EB, Choi KC. Roles of mesenchymal stem cells in tissue regeneration and immunomodulation. Biomol Ther 2019;27(1):25-33.

[42] Jackson WM, Nesti LJ, Tuan RS. Mesenchymal stem cell therapy for attenuation of scar formation during wound healing. Stem Cell Res Ther 2012;3(3):20. /pmc/articles/PMC3392767/

[43] Yates CC, Rodrigues M, Nuschke A, Johnson ZI, Whaley D, Stolz D, et al. Multipotent stromal cells/mesenchymal stem cells and fibroblasts combine to minimize skin hypertrophic scarring. Stem Cell Res Ther 2017;8(1):1-13.

[44] Domaszewska-Szostek A, Krzyżanowska M, Siemionow M. Cell-based therapies for chronic wounds tested in clinical studies: review. Ann Plast Surg 2019;83(6):e96-109. https://pubmed.ncbi.nlm.nih.gov/31335465/

[45] Liu J, Ren J, Su L, Cheng S, Zhou J, Ye X, et al. Human adipose tissue-derived stem cells inhibit the activity of keloid fibroblasts and fibrosis in a keloid model by paracrine signaling. Burns 2018;44(2):370-85. https://pubmed.ncbi.nlm.nih.gov/29029852/

[46] Han B, Fan J, Liu L, Tian J, Gan C, Yang Z, et al. Adipose-derived mesenchymal stem cells treatments for fibroblasts of fibrotic scar via downregulating TGF-β1 and Notch-1 expression enhanced by photobiomodulation therapy. Lasers Med Sci 2019;34(1). https://pubmed.ncbi.nlm.nih.gov/30367294/

[47] Fang F, Huang RL, Zheng Y, Liu M, Huo R. Bone marrow derived mesenchymal stem cells inhibit the proliferative and profibrotic phenotype of hypertrophic scar fibroblasts and keloid fibroblasts through paracrine signaling. J Dermatol Sci 2016;83(2):95-105. https://pubmed.ncbi.nlm.nih.gov/27211019/

[48] Sato C, Yamamoto Y, Funayama E, Furukawa H, Oyama A, Murao N, et al. Conditioned medium obtained from amnion-derived mesenchymal stem cell culture prevents activation of keloid fibroblasts. Plast Reconstr Surg 2018;141(2):390-8. https://pubmed.ncbi.nlm.nih.gov/29369991/

[49] Tooi M, Komaki M, Morioka C, Honda I, Iwasaki K, Yokoyama N, et al. Placenta mesenchymal stem cell derived exosomes confer plasticity on fibroblasts. J Cell Biochem 2016;117(7):1658-70. https://pubmed.ncbi.nlm.nih.gov/26640165/

[50] Hu L, Wang J, Zhou X, Xiong Z, Zhao J, Yu R, et al. Exosomes derived from human adipose mensenchymal stem cells accelerates cutaneous wound healing via optimizing the characteristics of fibroblasts. Sci Rep 2016;6:32993. https://pubmed.ncbi.nlm.nih.gov/27615560/

[51] Li M, Luan F, Zhao Y, Hao H, Liu J, Dong L, et al. Mesenchymal stem cell-conditioned medium accelerates wound healing with fewer scars. Int Wound J 2017;14(1):64-73. https://pubmed.ncbi.nlm.nih.gov/26635066/

[52] Pan C, Lang H, Zhang T, Wang R, Lin X, Shi P, et al. Conditioned medium derived from human amniotic stem cells delays H2O2-induced premature senescence in human dermal fibroblasts. Int J Mol Med 2019;44(5):1629-40.

https://pubmed.ncbi.nlm.nih.gov/31545472/

[53] Saheli M, Bayat M, Ganji R, Hendudari F, Kheirjou R, Pakzad M, et al. Human mesenchymal stem cells-conditioned medium improves diabetic wound healing mainly through modulating fibroblast behaviors. Arch Dermatol Res 2020;312(5):325-36. https://pubmed.ncbi.nlm.nih.gov/31786709/

[54] Li Y, Liu Z, Jin Y, Zhu X, Wang S, Yang J, et al. Differentiation of human amniotic mesenchymal stem cells into human anterior cruciate ligament fibroblast cells by in vitro coculture. Biomed Res Int 2017;2017. https://pubmed.ncbi.nlm.nih.gov/29085840/

[55] Straub JM, New J, Hamilton CD, Lominska C, Shnayder Y, Thomas SM. Radiation-induced fibrosis: mechanisms and implications for therapy. J Cancer Res Clin Oncol 2015;141(11):1985-94. https://link.springer.com/article/10.1007/s00432-015-1974-6

[56] Zhuang X mei, Zhou B. Exosome secreted by human gingival fibroblasts in radiation therapy inhibits osteogenic differentiation of bone mesenchymal stem cells by transferring miR-23a. Biomed Pharmacother 2020;131:110672. https://pubmed.ncbi.nlm.nih.gov/32889404/

[57] Kinane DF, Stathopoulou PG, Papapanou PN. Periodontal diseases. Nat Rev Dis Prim 2017;3:17038. https://pubmed.ncbi.nlm.nih.gov/28805207/

[58] Kaneda-Ikeda E, Iwata T, Mizuno N, Nagahara T, Kajiya M, Ouhara K, et al. Regulation of osteogenesis via miR-101-3p in mesenchymal stem cells by human gingival fibroblasts. J Bone Miner Metab 2020;38(4):442-55. https://pubmed.ncbi.nlm.nih.gov/31970478/

[59] Čamernik K, Mihelič A, Mihalič R, Haring G, Herman S, Marolt Presen D, et al. Comprehensive analysis of skeletal muscle- and bone-derived mesenchymal stem/stromal cells in patients with osteoarthritis and femoral neck fracture. Stem Cell Res Ther 2020;11(1):146. https://stemcellres.biomedcentral.com/articles/10.1186/s13287-020-01657-z

[60] Rosen CJ, Bouxsein ML. Mechanisms of disease: is osteoporosis the obesity of bone? Nat Clin Pract Rheumatol 2006;2(1):35-43. http://www.nature.com/doifinder/10.1038/ncprheum0070

[61] Pino AM, Rosen CJ, Rodríguez JP. In osteoporosis, differentiation of mesenchymal stem cells (MSCs) improves bone marrow adipogenesis. Biol Res 2012;45:279-87. http://www.scielo.cl/pdf/bres/v45n3/art09.pdf

[62] Smith LJ, Nerurkar NL, Choi KS, Harfe BD, Elliott DM. Degeneration and regeneration of the intervertebral disc: lessons from development. DMM Dis Model Mech 2011;4(1):31-41. https://pubmed.ncbi.nlm.nih.gov/21123625/

[63] Molinos M, Almeida CR, Caldeira J, Cunha C, Gonçalves RM, Barbosa MA. Inflammation in intervertebral disc degeneration and regeneration Vol. 12, Journal of the Royal Society Interface. Royal Society of London; 2015. /pmc/articles/PMC4345483/

[64] Ashinsky B, Smith HE, Mauck RL, Gullbrand SE. Intervertebral disc degeneration and regeneration: a motion segment perspective. Eur Cell Mater 2021;41:370-80. http://creativecommons.org/licenses/by-sa/4.0/

[65] Ural IH, Alptekin K, Ketenci A, Solakoglu S, Alpak H, Özyalçın S. Fibroblast transplantation results to the degenerated rabbit lumbar intervertebral discs. Open Orthop J 2017;11(1):404-16. https://pubmed.ncbi.nlm.nih.gov/28603572/

[66] Shi P, Chee A, Liu W, Chou PH, Zhu J, An HS. Therapeutic effects of cell therapy with neonatal human dermal fibroblasts and rabbit dermal fibroblasts on disc degeneration and inflammation. Spine J 2019;19(1):171-81. https://pubmed.ncbi.nlm.nih.gov/30142460/

[67] Borgström F, Karlsson L, Ortsäter G, Norton N, Halbout P, Cooper C, et al. Fragility fractures in Europe: burden, management and opportunities. Arch Osteoporos 2020;15(1):59. https://link.springer.com/article/10.1007%2Fs11657-020-0706-y

[68] Chang Y, Cho B, Kim S, Kim J. Direct conversion of fibroblasts to osteoblasts as a novel strategy for bone regeneration in elderly individuals Vol. 51, Experimental and Molecular Medicine 2019;51(5):54. https://pubmed.ncbi.nlm.nih.gov/31073120/

[69] Yamamoto K, Kishida T, Sato Y, Nishioka K, Ejima A, Fujiwara H, et al. Direct conversion of human fibroblasts into functional osteoblasts by defined factors. Proc Natl Acad Sci U S A 2015;112(19):6152-7. www.pnas.org/cgi/doi/10.1073/pnas.1420713112

[70] Bogdanowicz DR, Lu HH. Designing the stem cell microenvironment for guided connective tissue regeneration. Ann N Y Acad Sci 2017;1410(1):3-25.

[71] Matsuo Y, Saito T, Yamamoto A, Kohsaka H. Origins of fibroblasts in rheumatoid synovial tissues: implications from organ fibrotic models. Mod Rheumatol 2018;28(4):579-82. https://www.tandfonline.com/action/journalInformation?journalCode=imor20

[72] De Bari C. Are mesenchymal stem cells in rheumatoid arthritis the good or bad guys? Arthritis Res Ther 2015;17(1):1-9. https://arthritis-research.biomedcentral.com/articles/10.1186/s13075-015-0634-1

[73] El-Jawhari JJ, El-Sherbiny YM, Jones EA, McGonagle D. Mesenchymal stem cells, autoimmunity and rheumatoid arthritis. QJM 2014;107(7):505-14. /pmc/articles/PMC4071294/

[74] Rozier P, Maria A, Goulabchand R, Jorgensen C, Guilpain P, Noël D. Mesenchymal stem cells in systemic sclerosis: allogenic or autologous pproaches for therapeutic use? Front Immunol 2018;9:2938. www.frontiersin.org

[75] Rosa I, Romano E, Fioretto BS, Matucci-Cerinic M, Manetti M. Adipose-derived stem cells: Pathophysiologic implications vs therapeutic potential in systemic sclerosis. World J Stem Cells. 2021;13(1):30-48. https://www.wjgnet.com/1948-0210/full/v13/i1/30.htm

[76] Van SY, Noh YK, Kim SW, Oh YM, Kim IH, Park K. Human umbilical cord blood mesenchymal stem cells expansion via human fibroblast-derived matrix and their potentials toward regenerative application. Cell Tissue Res 2019;376(2):233-45. https://doi.org/10.1007/s00441-018-2971-2

[77] Sivan U, Jayakumar K, Krishnan LK. Matrix-directed differentiation of human adipose- derived mesenchymal stem cells to dermal-like fibroblasts that produce extracellular matrix. J Tissue Eng Regen Med 2016;10(10):E546-58. http://dx.doi.org/10.1016/j.trsl.2010.06.007

[78] Costa MHG, McDevitt TC, Cabral JMS, da Silva CL, Ferreira FC. Tridimensional configurations of human mesenchymal stem/stromal cells to enhance cell paracrine potential towards wound healing processes. J Biotechnol. 2017;262:28-39. https://www.sciencedirect.com/science/article/pii/S016816561731684X?via%3Dihub

[79] Engel P, Ranieri M, Felthaus O, Geis S, Haubner F, Aung T, et al. Effect

of HBO therapy on adipose-derived stem cells, fibroblasts and co-cultures: In vitro study of oxidative stress, angiogenic potential and production of pro-inflammatory growth factors in co-cultures. Clin Hemorheol Microcirc 2020;76(4):459-71. https://content.iospress.com/articles/clinical-hemorheology-and-microcirculation/ch209222

[80] Kim MH, Wu WH, Choi JH, Kim JH, Hong SH, Jun JH, et al. Conditioned medium from the three-dimensional culture of human umbilical cord perivascular cells accelerate the migration and proliferation of human keratinocyte and fibroblast. J Biomater Sci Polym Ed 2018;29(7-9):1066-80. https://pubmed.ncbi.nlm.nih.gov/28589787/

[81] Cerny MK, Hopfner U, Kirsch M, Haas EM, Wu F, Giunta R, et al. Occlusive dressing-induced secretomes influence the migration and proliferation of mesenchymal stem cells and fibroblasts differently. Eur J Med Res2018;23(1):60. https://pubmed.ncbi.nlm.nih.gov/30585140/

[82] Southworth TM, Naveen NB, Tauro TM, Leong NL, Cole BJ. The use of platelet-rich plasma in symptomatic knee osteoarthritis. J Knee Surg 2019;32(1):37-45. https://www.thieme-connect.com/products/ejournals/abstract/10.1055/s-0038-1675170

[83] Stessuk T, Puzzi MB, Chaim EA, Alves PCM, de Paula EV, Forte A, et al. Platelet-rich plasma (PRP) and adipose-derived mesenchymal stem cells: stimulatory effects on proliferation and migration of fibroblasts and keratinocytes in vitro. Arch Dermatol Res 2016;308(7):511-20. https://pubmed.ncbi.nlm.nih.gov/27394438/

[84] Ha SS, Song ES, Du P, Suhaeri M, Lee JH, Park K. Novel ECM patch combines poly(vinyl alcohol), human fibroblast-derived matrix, and mesenchymal stem cells for advanced wound healing. ACS Biomater Sci Eng 2020;6(7):4266-75. https://pubmed.ncbi.nlm.nih.gov/33463354/

[85] Steens J, Unger K, Klar L, Neureiter A, Wieber K, Hess J, et al. Direct conversion of human fibroblasts into therapeutically active vascular wall-typical mesenchymal stem cells. Cell Mol Life Sci 2020;77(17):3401-22. https://doi.org/10.1007/s00018-019-03358-0

[86] Lai PL, Lin H, Chen SF, Yang SC, Hung KH, Chang CF, et al. Efficient generation of chemically induced mesenchymal stem cells from human dermal fibroblasts. Sci Rep 2017;7:44534. https://pubmed.ncbi.nlm.nih.gov/28303927/

Section 2

Unique and Shared Fibroblast Mechanisms across Human Tissues and Pathologies

Chapter 3

The Role of Fibroblasts in Atherosclerosis Progression

Tadeja Kuret and Snežna Sodin-Šemrl

Abstract

The following chapter addresses vascular fibroblasts in a healthy, quiescent state, as well during vascular inflammation, focusing on atherosclerosis. The development of atherosclerosis, an inflammatory disease of medium- and large-sized arteries, has traditionally been viewed as an "inside-out" mechanism, with prominent roles of the innermost layer of the artery, consisting of endothelial cells. However, emerging evidence suggests a new paradigm of "outside-in" mechanism, including an earlier role for fibroblasts, constituents of the outermost adventitial layer of the artery. Phenotypic and functional changes of fibroblasts in adventitia may even occur prior to, or alongside endothelial activation. Activated adventitial fibroblasts, implicated in atherosclerosis progression, begin to transform into myofibroblasts, upregulate production of different proinflammatory cytokines, chemokines, growth factors, proteolytic enzymes, extracellular matrix proteins and reactive oxygen species, leading to extensive matrix remodeling, chemotaxis and recruitment of immune cells. Due to their suitable location for drug delivery systems, preventing fibroblast activation, modulating their activity or inducing myofibroblast dedifferentiation could represent a promising therapeutic approach for atherosclerosis regression.

Keywords: atherosclerosis, fibroblasts, inflammation, disease progression

1. Introduction

Fibroblasts are mesenchymal cells that are morphologically characterized as adherent, flat, elongated (spindle-shaped) cells with leveled, oval nuclei. One of their major roles is to produce and integrate structural proteins, such as collagen, elastin, and proteoglycans into the extracellular matrix (ECM) of most mesenchymal tissues and thus maintain their structural integrity [1].

In healthy arteries, fibroblasts can be found in the adventitia, the outermost layer of the vessel wall. Adventitial fibroblasts display numerous subtypes, even in a quiescent state, however, very little is known about their exact involvement in atherosclerosis development and progression [2]. Most of the attributed functions of adventitial fibroblasts have been largely extrapolated from findings describing fibroblasts in different tissues and organs, such as the skin. However, fibroblasts from different anatomic sites and tissues are functionally and phenotypically distinct. For example, cultured fetal and adult human skin fibroblasts derived from different anatomical sites expressed distinct transcriptional patterns of genes involved in extracellular matrix synthesis, lipid metabolism, and cell signaling pathways regulating proliferation, cell migration and fate determination [3].

IntechOpen

The discovered topographic differences of fibroblasts might be connected to the positional memory since adult fibroblast maintain key features of the HOX gene pattern expression, established during embryogenesis. Indeed, many HOX genes that encode a family of evolutionarily conserved transcription factors, are differentially expressed in fibroblasts derived from different anatomical sites, indicating that fibroblasts from each topographic site express a unique HOX gene expression pattern [3, 4].

Fibroblasts are metabolically active cells that play a central role in, not only matrix maintenance and remodeling and regulating ECM, but also in managing interstitial fluid volume and pressure, new tissue formation and wound healing. They have been found to be associated with many connective tissue pathologies, either due to their direct implication in the disease mechanism or due to the resulting fibrosis associated with damage in other cell types [5]. Recently, novel mechanisms proposed a prominent role of fibroblasts also in the development and progression of atherosclerosis. Atherosclerosis is a chronic, fibro-proliferative disease of the arterial vessel walls that underlies the development of many cardiovascular diseases (CVDs) and affects the structure and function of the involved arteries [6].

Vascular inflammation, leading to atherosclerosis, has been traditionally viewed as an "inside-out" response, beginning with the activation of endothelium and an inflammatory response that spreads outwards, from the intima towards media and adventitia, ultimately forming fibrous plaque and damaging all three vessel wall layers [7, 8]. The classical mechanism of atherogenesis has been challenged recently with emerging evidence supporting a new hypothesis of an "outside-in" mechanism, in which vascular inflammation actually begins in the adventitia and progresses inward towards the media and intima [8, 9], suggesting a more prominent role of fibroblasts than previously thought.

So, in order to pinpoint, the potential role of fibroblasts during atherosclerosis progression, we need to first look at the arterial wall composition and function.

2. Vessel wall structure and fibroblasts

2.1 Arterial vessel wall structure

Characterization of the resident, stromal cell populations and subpopulations in a blood vessel is an important step in understanding cellular contribution to vascular development and disease. Since atherosclerosis is prevalently a disease of large- and medium-sized arteries [10], we will focus here on the description of the structure of these vessels and corresponding vascular stromal cell populations.

The walls of large- and medium-sized arteries are a heterogeneous three-layered structure consisting of the tunica intima, media and adventitia. Each layer is unique in its histologic, biochemical and functional properties and is differentially involved in maintaining vascular homeostasis and regulating the vascular response to stress or injury [8]. The tunica intima or innermost layer represents a monolayer of endothelial cells, which are in direct contact with the blood flow. The intima is separated from the tunica media by a basement membrane and an internal elastic lamina. The tunica media consists of multiple layers of vascular smooth muscle cells (VSMC). The tunica adventitia or the outermost layer is separated from the media by an external elastic lamina and represents the most complex layer of the blood vessel [11]. The adventitia is composed primarily of fibroblasts in a loose connective tissue matrix, and it also contains resident immune cells (e.g. dendritic cells, macrophages, mast cells), pericytes, small blood vessels with endothelial cells (*vasa vasorum*), several progenitor cells and adrenergic nerve cells (**Figure 1**) [13].

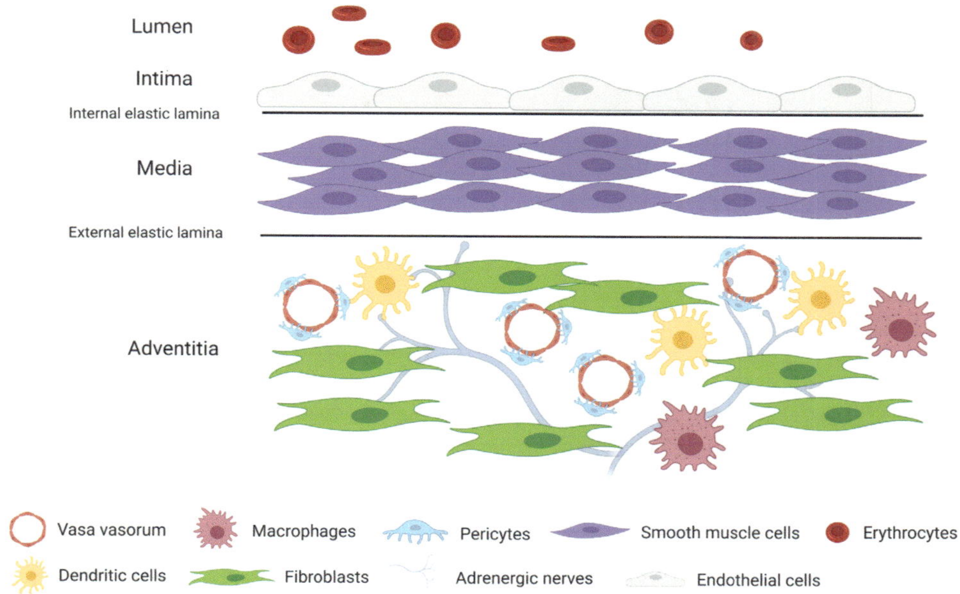

Figure 1.
Heterogeneous cellular composition of the vascular adventitia. Compared to arterial intima and media, which are composed of endothelial and smooth muscle cells, respectively, the arterial adventitia is composed of a variety of heterogeneous cell populations, including fibroblasts, immunomodulatory cells (e.g. dendritic cells, macrophages), vasa vasorum, *pericytes and adrenergic nerves. The figure was adapted from [12] and created using Biorender.*

For many years, adventitial cells were thought to have a limited physiological "static" function serving as structural support to the blood vessel, supplying oxygen and nutrients to the media of large vessels, and sustaining sympathetic innervation of the vessel wall [14]. However, latest *in vivo* and *in vitro* studies have shown that the adventitia represents a dynamic microenvironment that regulates both structural and functional properties of all three arterial layers [15]. The adventitia is an important source of cells that migrate towards the intima and media. For example, stem and progenitor cells that function and reside in the adventitia can transform into medial and intimal cells, such as VSMCs, and endothelial cells [16–18]. The adventitia of coronary arteries also contains cholinergic nerve terminals that release acetylcholine, diffusing to the intima layer of endothelium, where it induces the release of nitric oxide, causing VSMC relaxation and vasodilatation [19]. After stimulation with angiotensin II, adventitial fibroblasts can synthesize and release endothelin-1 (ET-1) that is important in mediating VSMC contraction [20]. The important role of adventitia is further supported by the role of *vasa vasorum* network, serving as a pipeline for inflammatory cell infiltration during vascular inflammation. In atherosclerosis, inflammation contributes to increased neovascularization and enhanced permeability of the adventitial *vasa vasorum*, allowing more inflammatory cells to enter the atherosclerotic plaque. Indeed, by suppressing the neovascularization of *vasa vasorum*, Moulton et al. [21] observed reduction in numbers of macrophages in atherosclerotic plaques and inhibition of atherosclerosis progression in experimental mice models [21]. Additionally, adventitial resident cells participate in initiation and regulation of vascular development, response to injury and tissue repair and thus, importantly contribute to disease development, especially intimal hyperplasia. This is mediated by their ability of responding to external physiological stress with intensive tissue repair or arterial remodeling [9, 16, 22]. Importantly, resident adventitial cells (e.g. fibroblasts) are often the first cells in the vascular wall to become activated in response to hormonal and inflammatory stimuli, as well as environmental stress, such as hypoxia/ischemia and hypertension [8, 15].

2.2 Fibroblasts in healthy arterial vessel walls

Understanding the role of fibroblasts in normal and pathologic conditions is often obstructed by the lack of reliable and specific markers. The fibroblast is therefore still one of the most difficult cell types to define *in vivo*, likely due to their heterogeneity (multiple subtypes) and plasticity [23].

In a healthy artery, adventitial fibroblasts are found in a non-active, quiescent state, and are usually defined by their location in the vessel wall since they can be separated from the more generally recognized smooth muscle cell layer by an external elastic lamina [24, 25]. All currently used markers to identify fibroblasts, including vimentin, platelet derived growth factor receptor α (PDGFRα), fibroblast specific protein 1 (FSP1), discoidin-domain receptor, and prolyl-4-hydroxylase, are potentially problematic, as they are also expressed in other cell types and are not present in all fibroblasts [3, 26, 27]. Therefore, to identify fibroblasts, investigators have to rely on the lack of markers for other cell lineages (e.g. non-lymphoid, non-endothelium, and non-epithelium), along with morphologic, functional, and biochemical characteristics [3].

Adventitial fibroblasts show differences in morphology, size, function and activity in the healthy, as well as stressed conditions or disease states [15]. For example, An et al. [28] found two major fibroblast subpopulations in the adventitia of rat thoracic aorta. The two populations were described as epithelioid-like cells and spindle-like cells, however only epithelioid-like fibroblasts were sensitive to stimulation with angiotensin II, a hormone involved in the development of hypertension and atherosclerosis [28]. Studying fibroblasts from the adventitia of bovine pulmonary artery, Das et al. [29] concluded that numerous phenotypically and biochemically distinct fibroblast subpopulations can be found and only a selective increase in the number of resident fibroblast subpopulations with enhanced growth capability was observed under hypoxic conditions [29].

With the development and increasing popularity of single cell RNA sequencing technology, it might now be possible to find markers, specific to adventitial fibroblasts, as well as to characterize in depth, their subpopulations in normal and diseased states [30]. Kalluri et al. [31] explored the cellular atlas of healthy mice aortas using single cell RNA sequencing. They showed that fibroblasts represent approximately 33% of all aortic cells and were defined by higher expression of PDGFRα and collagens/collagen-binding proteins (e.g. Col1a1, Col1a2, Dcn, Lum) whereas the expression of VSMC-associated contractile proteins (e.g. Myh11, Cnn1) was reduced. These fibroblasts clustered into two subpopulations and are probably derived from the adventitia, however their exact location needs to be confirmed by immunohistochemistry or in-situ hybridization [31]. Another study using the high resolution single cell analysis approach, was performed by Gu et al. [32] in aortic adventitial cells from wild type and apolipoprotein E-deficient (*ApoE-/-*) mice. They determined four heterogeneous mesenchymal populations with differential gene expression suggesting potential functions in ECM organization, immune regulation and bone formation. Furthermore, interaction of resident, mesenchymal cells with immune cells was enhanced in the adventitia of *ApoE-/-* mice. These data revealed a heterogeneous cellular landscape of the adventitia and confirmed fibroblast variability present already in the healthy, quiescent state [32].

3. Adventitial fibroblasts in vascular pathology

3.1 Contribution of adventitial fibroblasts to vascular pathology

In response to injury or environmental stress, adventitial fibroblasts can become activated, displaying altered phenotypic and functional properties. Activated fibroblasts intensely proliferate and increase production and deposition of ECM proteins, as well as proinflammatory cytokines, chemokines, adhesion molecules, matrix metalloproteinases (MMPs) and tissue inhibitors of MMPs (TIMPs), and growth factors, such as vascular endothelial growth factor (VEGF) [12, 33]. These molecules directly affect the phenotype of other resident cells in the vessel wall, such as VSMC and endothelial cells, promote neointima formation, regulate *vasa vasorum* expansion and affect the recruitment of infiltrating immune cells [8, 24]. Despite an excessive proliferation of activated fibroblasts, no hyperplasia of adventitia is usually observed in vascular pathologies. It is likely that many different mediators can also activate replication repressor signals in fibroblasts to limit or control replication. For instance, protein tyrosine phosphatases that regulate growth factor signaling in vascular remodeling, are upregulated in adventitial fibroblasts in response to vascular injury presumably to mitigate proliferative responses [34]. It was also demonstrated that adventitial fibroblasts under hypoxic conditions activate protein kinase C-zeta and MAPK phosphatase-1 that repress proliferative signals and limit the proliferation of fibroblasts [35, 36].

Vascular fibroblasts may also produce large amounts of reactive oxygen species (ROS) that seem to regulate their proliferation and ECM deposition [37, 38]. Activated fibroblasts increasingly interact with other cell types in the arterial wall, such as endothelial cells and VSMC and regulate their functions, as well as recruit immune cells into the vessel wall [39]. After their activation, some fibroblasts differentiate into myofibroblasts that contain bundles of stress fibers and can be identified by expression of contractile proteins, such as α-smooth muscle actin (αSMA). Multiple stimuli in the microenvironment, such as mechanical stress, growth factors (e.g. TGF-β), proinflammatory cytokines (e,g, IL-1β, IL-6, TNF-α), adhesion molecules, and ECM molecules can cause differentiation of a fibroblast towards the myofibroblast phenotype. Myofibroblasts contribute to extensive remodeling, intimal hyperplasia, and luminal stenosis due to their invasion and migration into the intima and increased production and secretion of ECM proteins [40–43].

The recognition that fibroblasts are not only able to generate, but also to sustain inflammatory responses, provides insight into why vascular inflammatory responses, in certain situations, fail to resolve. It is suggested that chronic inflammation occurs due to dysregulated fibroblast activity in which they fail to switch off their inflammatory programme, leading to the inappropriate survival and retention of leukocytes within inflamed tissue [44]. It is also clear that the activated adventitial fibroblasts play an important role in regulating *vasa vasorum* growth, which can contribute to ongoing vascular remodeling by acting as a conduit for delivery of inflammatory and progenitor cells [45].

Recent studies shed light on the implication of adventitial fibroblasts in different vascular pathologies, characterized by arterial remodeling and neointimal formation [43]. One of the most persistent findings in experimental *in vitro* and *in vivo* models is intensive adventitial remodeling, found very early in response to vascular injury or stress [46–48]. Adventitial remodeling in the vasculature has been characterized by increased proliferation of fibroblasts, which appear to be the first cells in the vessel wall that respond to different stimuli by their activation [49].

Direct evidence of fibroblast migration into the intima was provided in a study, performed by Li et al. [50], in which primary syngeneic adventitial fibroblasts were transduced with β-galactosidase (*LacZ*) and introduced into the adventitia of rat carotid arteries immediately after baloon injury. MRNA expression of *LacZ* and in situ enzymatic activity of β-galactosidase were detected in the media and the neo-intima, 7 days after injury. On the contrary, in the arteries that were not injured, the expression of *LacZ* and enzymatic activity of β-galactosidase were restricted to the adventitia [50]. Similar findings were later reported by Han et al. [51] showing that adventitial fibroblasts migrated to the media and intima on seventh day after balloon injury in the rat carotid artery. The results were obtained by direct labeling of adventitial fibroblasts using *in vivo* gene transfer technique, as well as transmission electron microscopy [51]. Furthermore, Dutzmann et al. [52] discovered that early activation of adventitial fibroblasts after wire-induced injury in C57BL/6 mice stimulated their proliferation and release of proinflammatory cytokines and growth factors, and the subsequent proliferation of VSMC, resulting in neointima formation [52].

Pulmonary artery hypertension (PAH) is one of the vascular pathologies, characterized by extensive arterial remodeling and neointima formation, in which fibroblasts were shown to play an important role [53]. For example, in the neonatal bovine hypoxic PAH model, adventitial fibroblasts were found to undergo the earliest and most significant increases in proliferation, among all the vascular wall cell types [54]. Fibroblasts derived from experimental hypoxia-induced PAH and patients with PAH, display a hyperproliferative, apoptosis-resistant, and proinflammatory phenotype, defined by increased production of IL-6, IL-1β, CCL2/MCP1, CCL12/SDF1, VCAM1 and osteopontin [12, 55]. Moreover, when naïve bone marrow derived macrophages were exposed *in vitro* to conditioned medium generated by adventitial fibroblasts from human PAH patients and hypoxia induced PAH animals, they increased the transcription of several markers of activation (e.g. Cd163, Cd206, Il4ra and Socs3) [56]. These findings suggest that activated adventitial fibroblasts in PAH secrete various soluble factors required for macrophage activation and polarization leading to the propagation of inflammation from adventitia towards media and intima, supporting the "outside-in" hypothesis [53].

3.2 The role of fibroblasts in atherosclerosis and potential fibroblast-targeted therapy

Several findings suggest a role of fibroblasts in all stages of atherosclerosis, from initial phase to fibrous cap and plaque formation. It is becoming evident that adventitial cells, including adventitial fibroblasts are one of the first cells to respond to injury and become activated in the initial stage of atherosclerosis, even before the formation of atherosclerotic lesions, supporting the new "outside-in" hypothesis [46, 48].

Studies have shown that in various presentations of CVDs, the adventitia becomes heavily populated with multiple immune cell types, including monocytes, macrophages and T-cells, while adventitial fibroblasts proliferate increasingly and differentiate into myofibroblasts [33, 57–59]. Furthermore, several studies reported on increased *vasa vasorum* neovascularization in early atherosclerosis prior to the development of endothelial dysfunction [60, 61]. Neovascularization may act as a pipeline, allowing the entry of immune cells into the site of injury, as the density of *vasa vasorum* is highly correlated with the extent of inflammatory infiltrates in *ApoE-/-* mice [21]. These studies indicate that increased neovascularization of *vasa vasorum* in adventitia, that promotes inflammatory response and plaque angiogenesis, can occur before the endothelial activation and dysfunction in the intima [8]. Adventitial fibroblasts can regulate the growth and neovascularization of *vasa vasorum* through the release of soluble angiogenic growth factors, such as VEGF, TGF-β and platelet-derived growth factor (PDGF). Furthermore, with the release of chemokines, such as monocyte chemoattractant protein (MCP1), fibroblasts facilitate infiltration of circulating leukocytes, further increasing the growth of the *vasa vasorum* and perpetuating the inflammatory response [37].

Xu et al. [62] investigated the role of adventitial fibroblasts in atherosclerotic lesion formation by comparing the characteristics of adventitial fibroblasts from *ApoE-/-* and wild type mice. They found αSMA expressing adventitial fibroblast in *ApoE-/-* mice, but not in wild type mice. The gene expression of collagen I and collagen III was upregulated in adventitial fibroblasts from *ApoE-/-* mice, compared to the wild type mice. Furthermore, adventitial fibroblasts from *ApoE-/-* mice synthesized more TGF-β, MCP1, and PDGFβ and exhibited proliferatory and migratory properties [62]. MCP1 is important in regulation of migration and infiltration of monocytes into the vessel wall, which differentiate into macrophages, form foam cells and importantly contribute to fatty streak formation [63]. The effects of adventitial fibroblasts are also ascribed to ROS produced by adventitial fibroblast NADPH oxidases that play important roles in neointimal formation and growth in vascular pathologies, including atherosclerosis [37]. Xu et al. [64] studied ROS production and expression of NADPH oxidase subunit p47phox in the hyperlipid diet-induced atherosclerosis in the *ApoE-/-* mouse model. The activated fibroblasts from aortas of *ApoE-/-* mice displayed upregulated NADPH oxidase activity, augmented ROS production, and increased p47phox levels, compared with wild-type mice. ROS production was also associated with the increased proliferation and migration of adventitial fibroblasts. In addition, silencing of p47phox decreased the proliferation and migration of fibroblasts from *ApoE-/-* mice [64]. Fibroblasts, in response to ROS proliferate and release a number of growth factors and other mediators that influence vascular function, including ET1, PDGF, endothelial growth factor (EGF), fibroblast growth factor2 (FGF2), prostaglandin H2 (PGH2), and cyclophilins [65, 66]. In addition, ROS can also stimulate phenotypic switch of VSMC from the contractile to the proliferative and migratory one, suggesting that fibroblasts can indirectly influence other cell types inside the vessel wall [38].

In the initial phase of fibrosis, injured arteries start with tissue remodeling, and the formation of initial fibrous plaque actually represents a protective process; however, as in all chronic inflammatory conditions, fibrotic components in the plaque produce surplus levels of cytokines and proteolytic enzymes, causing excessive remodeling and tissue damage [59]. In advanced stages of atherosclerosis, fibrosis plays a central role and fibroblasts are the major cell population involved in remodeling of ECM in the fibrous plaque [59]. The most important functions of fibroblasts in progressed atherosclerosis include regulation of the inflammatory response, ECM protein production, and maintenance of the structural integrity of the plaque as well as regulated balance of MMP production, to enable beneficial tissue remodeling, alongside preventing plaque rupture, for instance [59, 67]. The potential role of fibroblasts in the development of atherosclerosis is shown in **Figure 2**.

Regulation of fibroblasts activities might be beneficial in controlling or reversing the progression of atherosclerosis, hence, the adventitial fibroblast may be an attractive target for therapeutic intervention. Furthermore, the location of the adventitia as the outermost arterial layer makes it suitable for drug delivery and gene therapy [24]. It has already been shown that local adventitial drug delivery into coronary arteries results in better efficiency compared to luminal or intimal delivery methods [71]. Low efficiency of gene transfer to cells in adventitia by intraluminal administration has been reported and efficient transfection of these

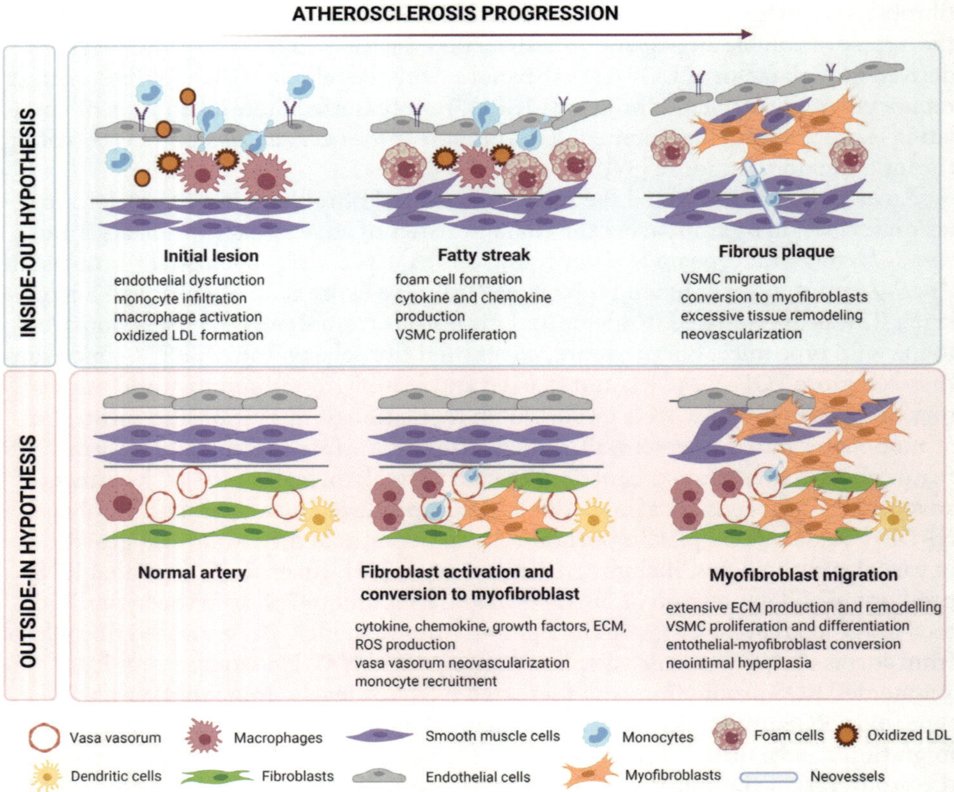

Figure 2.
The potential role of fibroblasts during atherosclerosis progression. Emerging evidence suggests that adventitial fibroblasts are activated in the initial stage of atherosclerosis, supporting the new "outside-in" hypothesis, which proposes that vascular inflammation begins in the adventitia and progresses inward towards the media and intima. In contrast, the original "inside-out" hypothesis of atherosclerosis proposes that the inflammatory response spreads from the intima outward towards adventitia with a more prominent role of endothelial and smooth muscle cells. The figure was adapted from [68–70] and created using Biorender. Legend: ECM, extracellular matrix; LDL, low density lipoprotein; ROS, reactive oxygen species; VSMC, vascular smooth muscle cells.

cells is achieved only when endothelium is denuded or damaged. In atherosclerotic arteries, intimal hyperplasia might present an additional barrier for intraluminal delivery. To overcome these problems, delivery from the adventitial side might be considered. On the other hand, numerous attempts to transfect or deliver the therapeutic agents to the media from the adventitial side of large blood vessels have failed because of the impenetrable nature of the external elastic lamina, separating adventitia from the media layer. This barrier hence allows for selective adventitial delivery and specific targeting of cells residing in adventitia [72].

Perivascular delivery of an adenoviral vector expressing a NADPH oxidase inhibitor in the rat carotid artery adventitia significantly reduced neointimal formation after balloon angioplasty. This specific vector targeted adventitial fibroblasts, and it did not affect VSMC in the media [73]. Targeting proteins, expressed by activated fibroblasts could attenuate vascular inflammatory responses and ameliorate vascular disease, including atherosclerosis. Recently, it was discovered that inhibition of expression or activity of fibroblast activation protein (FAP), that is expressed in activated but not in quiescent fibroblasts and was found to be associated with atherosclerotic plaques, can attenuate progression of atherosclerosis by increasing plaque stability in experimental mice models of atherosclerosis [74].

Reports on animal models of cardiomyopathy have indicated that reversibility of fibrosis was possible, with losartan (a selective angiotensin II type 1 receptor antagonist), which suppressed TGF-β expression [75, 76]. However, angiotensin II type 1 receptor is expressed also on VSMC and TGF-β can be produced by multiple cell types, in addition to fibroblasts.

A substantial number of adventitial fibroblasts can differentiate into myofibroblasts during initial stages of atherosclerosis, upon the influence of proinflammatory cytokines, chemokines adhesion molecules, growth factors and ECM proteins [33, 77]. For example, TGF-β induces the transition of a fibroblast into the myofibroblast by stimulating αSMA expression and collagen production [41, 42]. These highly proliferative αSMA-positive cells were found to be widely distributed in atherosclerotic plaques [24]. However, myofibroblasts in the atherosclerotic plaques can derive from multiple other sources, including VSMC [39], the endothelial to mesenchymal transition [78], as well as resident macrophages [79] (**Figure 3**). Myofibroblasts can contribute to changes in the function and structure of the vessel wall that occur during atherosclerosis (i.e arterial remodeling) due to their contractile properties and enhanced ECM protein production [80]. Myofibroblasts migrate from the adventitia to the media and intima and contribute to intimal hyperplasia [81, 82].

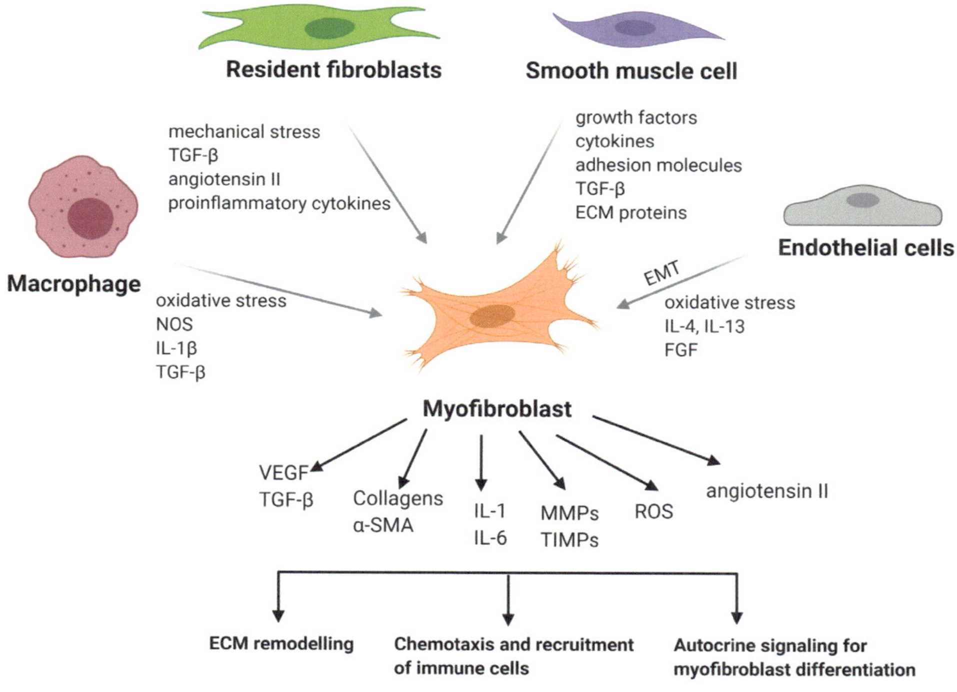

Figure 3.
Various cells from the arterial wall can differentiate into myofibroblasts in atherosclerosis. Macrophages, resident fibroblasts, smooth muscle cells and endothelial cells can differentiate into myofibroblasts, depending on tissue microenvironment and inflammatory mediators. Myofibroblasts are characterized by increased expression of α-smooth muscle actin and synthesize and release large amounts of ECM proteins, growth factors, proinflammatory cytokines, proteolytic enzymes and their inhibitors, as well as reactive oxygen species. They are responsible for extensive ECM remodeling, increased chemotaxis and recruitment of immune cells and provide signals for further myofibroblast differentiation. The figure was adapted from [41] and created using Biorender. Legend: αSMA: α-smooth muscle actin; ECM: extracellular matrix; EMT, endothelial mesenchymal transition FGF: fibroblast growth factor; IL: interleukin; NOS: nitric oxide synthase; MMPs: matrix metalloproteases; ROS: reactive oxygen species; TGF-β: transforming growth factor-β; TIMPs: tissue inhibitors of MMPs; VEGF: vascular endothelial growth factor.

Although myofibroblasts were previously considered to be terminally differentiated cells, their capacity for dedifferentiation, defined as the loss of αSMA, is now well recognized and necessary to resolve idiopathic pulmonary fibrosis [83]. Several factors, such as prostaglandin E2 (PGE2), nuclear factor erythroid 2-related factor2 (Nrf2) and FGFs have shown the ability to dedifferentiate established lung and corneal myofibroblasts and might be promising therapeutic targets also for adventitial myofibroblasts in atherosclerosis [84]. For example, treatment with PGE2 was shown to inhibit proliferation and collagen I expression in fibroblasts extracted from histologically normal lung tissue [85]. In TGF-β or ET-1-activated lung myofibroblasts, treatment with PGE2 induced a dose-dependent decrease in αSMA and collagen I expression that was associated with inhibition of focal adhesion kinase signaling [86]. Sulforaphane, a Nrf2 activator, induced myofibroblast dedifferentiation in cultured lung fibroblasts from patients with idiopathic pulmonary fibrosis, as well as inhibited TGF-β-mediated profibrotic effects [87]. Corneal myofibroblasts that were grown in the presence of FGF1 or FGF2 and heparin reduced expression of αSMA, TGF-β receptors, and cadherins, thus promoting the quiescent fibroblast phenotype [88]. FGF21 has been shown to induce angiotensin-converting enzyme 2 (ACE2), and thus inhibit vascular remodeling, hypertension and fibrosis, and when stimulating with adiponectin, FGF21 may inhibit aortic inflammation in atherosclerosis, as well as decrease cardiac dysfunction in myocardial infarction, attenuate smooth muscle cell proliferation and migration and lower macrophage oxidizes low-density lipoprotein uptake [89]. In addition, Fgf21 knock-out mice have been reported to show impaired lipid metabolism [90]. So, FGF21 has shown promise, as a potential therapeutic for atherosclerosis, but would need further investigation in regard to its effects on leukocytes and activities of its receptors.

3.3 The origin of fibroblasts in atherosclerosis

Fibroblast heterogeneity in quiescent and diseased state might be a result of their various origins, as well as plasticity, since they can transform into different cell types, subsequently to their adaptation to stress or injury. Evidence suggests that fibroblasts involved in atherosclerosis may originate from different adventitial mesenchymal stem/progenitor cells, however, recent studies revealed they can also originate from VSMC or endothelial cells [30].

Several distinct progenitor/stem cell populations with the capacity to differentiate into endothelial cells, VSMC, fibroblasts, and macrophages reside in a specialized niche in the adventitia at the media-adventitia border [91]. A population of vascular progenitor cells in the aortic adventitia of *ApoE−/−* mice expressing the stem cell markers Sca1 and CD34 was described that might differentiate to vascular fibroblasts [92]. However, the exact identity of adventitial progenitor/stem cells is still controversial, since fibroblast also have the ability to acquire stem cell properties by upregulating Sca1 [93–95]. Moreover, mesenchymal stem cells and fibroblasts are similar in terms of morphology and share the expression of a number of surface markers, such as CD90, CD73, CD105, vimentin and FSP1. Some researchers therefore suggest that these adventitial stem cells positive for Sca1 are actually fibroblasts [30, 93]. For example, Tang et al. [96] showed that 40% of Sca1-positive adventitial stem cells also express PDGFRα, found to be expressed on the surface of fibroblasts [96]. Using single cell RNA sequencing, Gu et al. [32] identified four mesenchymal clusters in the aortas of *ApoE−/−*, as well as wild type mice, but did not annotate them as stem or progenitor cells. However, one of the clusters displayed high expression of Sca1 indicating stem cell properties [32]. The separation between adventitial fibroblasts and progenitor/stem cells seem to be much smaller than previously thought and cell transition of stem cells into fibroblasts or vice versa appears to be common in atherosclerosis [30]. It would be interesting to further investigate how this transdifferentiation would affect the pathological process of atherosclerosis and whether it could be targeted to reverse atherosclerosis progression.

The evidence that fibroblasts might originate from VSMC came from Wirka et al. in 2019 [97]. They reported that VSMC can transform into fibroblast-like cells (termed "fibromyocytes"), found in the arteries of *ApoE−/−* mice, as well as atherosclerotic human coronary arteries. Fibromyocytes expressed lower levels of VSMC differentiation markers and increased expression of genes, associated with fibroblast cluster, such as lumican, decorin and biglycan. However, fibromyocytes were transcriptionally different from the fibroblasts indicating that either they will further dedifferentiate into fibroblasts or they might represent another distinct population of fibroblasts [97]. Furthermore, it is currently still unclear, whether fibroblasts might also transform into VSMC.

Endothelial cells can serve as a possible source of atherosclerotic fibroblasts since they can undergo endothelial-mesenchymal transition, promoting atherosclerosis progression [98]. This was elegantly shown in 2016 by Evrard et al. [78] using a tamoxifen-inducible endothelial lineage tracking system in *ApoE−/−* mice. After 8 weeks of high fat diet, the mouse atherosclerotic plaques consisted of one third endothelial-derived cells positive for FAP and a range of other fibroblast markers. These cells further expanded in number in advanced atherosclerotic plaques. *In vitro* modeling confirmed that endothelial-mesenchymal transition is driven by TGF-β signaling, oxidative stress and hypoxia that are all characteristic for atherosclerosis. Furthermore, the extent of this transition correlated with an unstable plaque phenotype in humans, driven by altered collagen and MMP production that might be associated with clinical events [78].

Whether functional differences between fibroblasts, originating from different sources exist and what is their exact contribution to development and/or progression of atherosclerosis, still remain two important and open questions.

4. Conclusions

Recently, the well-established "inside-out" hypothesis of atherosclerotic development and progression has been revitalized to involve an "outside-in" component, including an earlier role for fibroblasts in the tunica adventitia layer. It is now thought that early "outside-in" events, with more prominent roles of fibroblasts in adventitia may even occur prior to, or alongside endothelial activation. Adventitial fibroblasts involved in atherosclerosis comprise a very heterogeneous population, due to their differential origins (mesenchymal stem/progenitor cells, smooth muscle cells, endothelial cells, macrophages) and an extensive repertoire of possible cell transitions into αSMA^+ myofibroblasts, or even back to stem cells. It is thought that when resident fibroblasts begin to transform into αSMA^+ myofibroblasts, this allows for intense release of VEGF, TGF-β, collagens, IL-1, IL-6, MMPs, ROS and angiotensin II, among other factors, that could lead to perpetual autocrine differentiation and inflammatory, proliferative states, responsible for ECM remodeling, chemotaxis and recruitment of immune cells. Their heterogeneity and consequently, a general lack of specific markers, both contribute to difficulties in studying their exact phenotypes and functions in atherosclerosis. The recent development and accessibility of single cell RNA sequencing technology provides new opportunities to find answers to the remaining questions in an unbiased manner. Furthermore, modulating fibroblast activity, preventing their activation or inducing myofibroblast dedifferentiation in atherosclerotic arteries could represent a promising therapeutic approach for atherosclerosis regression. The plasticity of the atherosclerotic plaque may reform and dynamically remodel many times, before either rupturing or, on the other hand, stabilizing with a plaque cap or even regressing, depending on, among many factors, also molecules in the microenvironment (micro-exoproteome) and presence of certain cellular profiles that may help lean the process either way.

Conflict of interest

The authors declare no conflict of interest.

Author details

Tadeja Kuret[1,2] and Snežna Sodin-Šemrl[2,3*]

1 Institute of Cell Biology, Faculty of Medicine, University of Ljubljana, Slovenia

2 FAMNIT, University of Primorska, Koper, Slovenia

3 Department of Rheumatology, University Medical Centre Ljubljana, Slovenia

*Address all correspondence to: ssodin1@yahoo.com

References

[1] Lynch MD, Watt FM. Fibroblast heterogeneity: implications for human disease. J Clin Invest. 2018;128(1): 26-35.

[2] Di Wang H, Ratsep MT, Chapman A, Boyd R. Adventitial fibroblasts in vascular structure and function: the role of oxidative stress and beyond. Can J Physiol Pharmacol. 2010;88(3):177-86.

[3] Chang HY, Chi JT, Dudoit S, Bondre C, van de Rijn M, Botstein D, et al. Diversity, topographic differentiation, and positional memory in human fibroblasts. Proc Natl Acad Sci U S A. 2002;99(20):12877-82.

[4] Rinn JL, Wang JK, Allen N, Brugmann SA, Mikels AJ, Liu H, et al. A dermal HOX transcriptional program regulates site-specific epidermal fate. Genes Dev. 2008;22(3):303-7.

[5] McAnulty RJ. Fibroblasts and myofibroblasts: their source, function and role in disease. Int J Biochem Cell Biol. 2007;39(4):666-71.

[6] Schaftenaar F, Frodermann V, Kuiper J, Lutgens E. Atherosclerosis: the interplay between lipids and immune cells. Curr Opin Lipidol. 2016;27(3): 209-15.

[7] Libby P, Buring JE, Badimon L, Hansson GK, Deanfield J, Bittencourt MS, et al. Atherosclerosis. Nat Rev Dis Primers. 2019;5(1):56.

[8] Maiellaro K, Taylor WR. The role of the adventitia in vascular inflammation. Cardiovasc Res. 2007;75(4):640-8.

[9] Sartore S, Chiavegato A, Faggin E, Franch R, Puato M, Ausoni S, et al. Contribution of adventitial fibroblasts to neointima formation and vascular remodeling: from innocent bystander to active participant. Circ Res. 2001;89(12):1111-21.

[10] Yurdagul A, Jr., Finney AC, Woolard MD, Orr AW. The arterial microenvironment: the where and why of atherosclerosis. Biochem J. 2016;473(10):1281-95.

[11] Milutinovic A, Suput D, Zorc-Pleskovic R. Pathogenesis of atherosclerosis in the tunica intima, media, and adventitia of coronary arteries: An updated review. Bosn J Basic Med Sci. 2020;20(1):21-30.

[12] Stenmark KR, Yeager ME, El Kasmi KC, Nozik-Grayck E, Gerasimovskaya EV, Li M, et al. The adventitia: essential regulator of vascular wall structure and function. Annu Rev Physiol. 2013;75:23-47.

[13] Sorrell JM, Caplan AI. Fibroblasts-a diverse population at the center of it all. Int Rev Cell Mol Biol. 2009;276:161-214.

[14] Nava E, Llorens S. The Local Regulation of Vascular Function: From an Inside-Outside to an Outside-Inside Model. Front Physiol. 2019;10:729.

[15] Tinajero MG, Gotlieb AI. Recent Developments in Vascular Adventitial Pathobiology: The Dynamic Adventitia as a Complex Regulator of Vascular Disease. Am J Pathol. 2020;190(3): 520-34.

[16] Chen Y, Wong MM, Campagnolo P, Simpson R, Winkler B, Margariti A, et al. Adventitial stem cells in vein grafts display multilineage potential that contributes to neointimal formation. Arterioscler Thromb Vasc Biol. 2013;33(8):1844-51.

[17] Passman JN, Dong XR, Wu SP, Maguire CT, Hogan KA, Bautch VL, et al. A sonic hedgehog signaling domain in the arterial adventitia supports resident Sca1+ smooth muscle progenitor cells. Proc Natl Acad Sci U S A. 2008;105(27):9349-54.

[18] Zengin E, Chalajour F, Gehling UM, Ito WD, Treede H, Lauke H, et al. Vascular wall resident progenitor cells: a source for postnatal vasculogenesis. Development. 2006;133(8): 1543-51.

[19] Gutterman DD. Adventitia-dependent influences on vascular function. Am J Physiol. 1999;277(4): H1265-72.

[20] Di Wang H, Hope S, Du Y, Quinn MT, Cayatte A, Pagano PJ, et al. Paracrine role of adventitial superoxide anion in mediating spontaneous tone of the isolated rat aorta in angiotensin II-induced hypertension. Hypertension. 1999;33(5):1225-32.

[21] Moulton KS, Vakili K, Zurakowski D, Soliman M, Butterfield C, Sylvin E, et al. Inhibition of plaque neovascularization reduces macrophage accumulation and progression of advanced atherosclerosis. Proc Natl Acad Sci U S A. 2003;100(8): 4736-41.

[22] Stenmark KR, Nozik-Grayck E, Gerasimovskaya E, Anwar A, Li M, Riddle S, et al. The adventitia: Essential role in pulmonary vascular remodeling. Compr Physiol. 2011;1(1):141-61.

[23] Di Carlo SE, Peduto L. The perivascular origin of pathological fibroblasts. J Clin Invest. 2018;128(1): 54-63.

[24] Kuwabara JT, Tallquist MD. Tracking Adventitial Fibroblast Contribution to Disease: A Review of Current Methods to Identify Resident Fibroblasts. Arterioscler Thromb Vasc Biol. 2017;37(9):1598-607.

[25] Michel JB, Thaunat O, Houard X, Meilhac O, Caligiuri G, Nicoletti A. Topological determinants and consequences of adventitial responses to arterial wall injury. Arterioscler Thromb Vasc Biol. 2007;27(6):1259-68.

[26] Matsuyama W, Watanabe M, Shirahama Y, Mitsuyama H, Higashimoto I, Osame M, et al. Discoidin domain receptor 1 contributes to the survival of lung fibroblast in idiopathic pulmonary fibrosis. Am J Pathol. 2006;168(3):866-77.

[27] Goodpaster T, Legesse-Miller A, Hameed MR, Aisner SC, Randolph-Habecker J, Coller HA. An immunohistochemical method for identifying fibroblasts in formalin-fixed, paraffin-embedded tissue. J Histochem Cytochem. 2008;56(4): 347-58.

[28] An SJ, Liu P, Shao TM, Wang ZJ, Lu HG, Jiao Z, et al. Characterization and functions of vascular adventitial fibroblast subpopulations. Cell Physiol Biochem. 2015;35(3):1137-50.

[29] Das M, Dempsey EC, Reeves JT, Stenmark KR. Selective expansion of fibroblast subpopulations from pulmonary artery adventitia in response to hypoxia. Am J Physiol Lung Cell Mol Physiol. 2002;282(5):L976-86.

[30] Tillie R, van Kuijk K, Sluimer JC. Fibroblasts in atherosclerosis: heterogeneous and plastic participants. Curr Opin Lipidol. 2020;31(5):273-8.

[31] Kalluri AS, Vellarikkal SK, Edelman ER, Nguyen L, Subramanian A, Ellinor PT, et al. Single-Cell Analysis of the Normal Mouse Aorta Reveals Functionally Distinct Endothelial Cell Populations. Circulation. 2019;140(2):147-63.

[32] Gu W, Ni Z, Tan YQ, Deng J, Zhang SJ, Lv ZC, et al. Adventitial Cell Atlas of wt (Wild Type) and ApoE (Apolipoprotein E)-Deficient Mice Defined by Single-Cell RNA Sequencing. Arterioscler Thromb Vasc Biol. 2019;39(6):1055-71.

[33] Coen M, Gabbiani G, Bochaton-Piallat ML. Myofibroblast-

mediated adventitial remodeling: an underestimated player in arterial pathology. Arterioscler Thromb Vasc Biol. 2011;31(11):2391-6.

[34] Micke P, Hackbusch D, Mercan S, Stawowy P, Tsuprykov O, Unger T, et al. Regulation of tyrosine phosphatases in the adventitia during vascular remodelling. Biochem Biophys Res Commun. 2009;382(4):678-84.

[35] Das M, Bouchey DM, Moore MJ, Hopkins DC, Nemenoff RA, Stenmark KR. Hypoxia-induced proliferative response of vascular adventitial fibroblasts is dependent on g protein-mediated activation of mitogen-activated protein kinases. J Biol Chem. 2001;276(19):15631-40.

[36] Short MD, Fox SM, Lam CF, Stenmark KR, Das M. Protein kinase Czeta attenuates hypoxia-induced proliferation of fibroblasts by regulating MAP kinase phosphatase-1 expression. Mol Biol Cell. 2006;17(4):1995-2008.

[37] Haurani MJ, Pagano PJ. Adventitial fibroblast reactive oxygen species as autacrine and paracrine mediators of remodeling: bellwether for vascular disease? Cardiovasc Res. 2007;75(4): 679-89.

[38] Rey FE, Pagano PJ. The reactive adventitia: fibroblast oxidase in vascular function. Arterioscler Thromb Vasc Biol. 2002;22(12):1962-71.

[39] Hu D, Yin C, Luo S, Habenicht AJR, Mohanta SK. Vascular Smooth Muscle Cells Contribute to Atherosclerosis Immunity. Front Immunol. 2019;10:1101.

[40] Li N, Cheng W, Huang T, Yuan J, Wang X, Song M. Vascular Adventitia Calcification and Its Underlying Mechanism. PLoS One. 2015;10(7):e0132506.

[41] Serini G, Gabbiani G. Mechanisms of myofibroblast activity and phenotypic modulation. Exp Cell Res. 1999;250(2):273-83.

[42] Powell DW, Mifflin RC, Valentich JD, Crowe SE, Saada JI, West AB. Myofibroblasts. I. Paracrine cells important in health and disease. Am J Physiol. 1999;277(1):C1-9.

[43] Enzerink A, Vaheri A. Fibroblast activation in vascular inflammation. J Thromb Haemost. 2011;9(4):619-26.

[44] Buckley CD, Pilling D, Lord JM, Akbar AN, Scheel-Toellner D, Salmon M. Fibroblasts regulate the switch from acute resolving to chronic persistent inflammation. Trends Immunol. 2001;22(4):199-204.

[45] Stenmark KR, Frid MG, Yeager M, Li M, Riddle S, McKinsey T, et al. Targeting the adventitial microenvironment in pulmonary hypertension: A potential approach to therapy that considers epigenetic change. Pulm Circ. 2012;2(1):3-14.

[46] Wang J, Wang Y, Wang J, Guo X, Chan EC, Jiang F. Adventitial Activation in the Pathogenesis of Injury-Induced Arterial Remodeling: Potential Implications in Transplant Vasculopathy. Am J Pathol. 2018; 188(4):838-45.

[47] Stenmark KR, Davie N, Frid M, Gerasimovskaya E, Das M. Role of the adventitia in pulmonary vascular remodeling. Physiology (Bethesda). 2006;21:134-45.

[48] Goel SA, Guo LW, Liu B, Kent KC. Mechanisms of post-intervention arterial remodelling. Cardiovasc Res. 2012;96(3):363-71.

[49] McGrath JC, Deighan C, Briones AM, Shafaroudi MM, McBride M, Adler J, et al. New aspects of vascular remodelling: the involvement of all vascular cell types. Exp Physiol. 2005;90(4):469-75.

[50] Li G, Chen SJ, Oparil S, Chen YF, Thompson JA. Direct in vivo evidence demonstrating neointimal migration of adventitial fibroblasts after balloon injury of rat carotid arteries. Circulation. 2000;101(12):1362-5.

[51] Han X, Wu A, Wang J, Chang H, Zhao Y, Zhang Y, et al. Activation and Migration of Adventitial Fibroblasts Contributes to Vascular Remodeling. Anat Rec (Hoboken). 2018;301(7): 1216-23.

[52] Dutzmann J, Koch A, Weisheit S, Sonnenschein K, Korte L, Haertle M, et al. Sonic hedgehog-dependent activation of adventitial fibroblasts promotes neointima formation. Cardiovasc Res. 2017;113(13):1653-63.

[53] Hu Y, Chi L, Kuebler WM, Goldenberg NM. Perivascular Inflammation in Pulmonary Arterial Hypertension. Cells. 2020;9(11).

[54] Belknap JK, Orton EC, Ensley B, Tucker A, Stenmark KR. Hypoxia increases bromodeoxyuridine labeling indices in bovine neonatal pulmonary arteries. Am J Respir Cell Mol Biol. 1997;16(4):366-71.

[55] Li M, Riddle SR, Frid MG, El Kasmi KC, McKinsey TA, Sokol RJ, et al. Emergence of fibroblasts with a proinflammatory epigenetically altered phenotype in severe hypoxic pulmonary hypertension. J Immunol. 2011;187(5):2711-22.

[56] El Kasmi KC, Pugliese SC, Riddle SR, Poth JM, Anderson AL, Frid MG, et al. Adventitial fibroblasts induce a distinct proinflammatory/profibrotic macrophage phenotype in pulmonary hypertension. J Immunol. 2014;193(2):597-609.

[57] Campbell KA, Lipinski MJ, Doran AC, Skaflen MD, Fuster V, McNamara CA. Lymphocytes and the adventitial immune response in atherosclerosis. Circ Res. 2012;110(6): 889-900.

[58] Rademakers T, van der Vorst EP, Daissormont IT, Otten JJ, Theodorou K, Theelen TL, et al. Adventitial lymphatic capillary expansion impacts on plaque T cell accumulation in atherosclerosis. Sci Rep. 2017;7:45263.

[59] Singh S, Torzewski M. Fibroblasts and Their Pathological Functions in the Fibrosis of Aortic Valve Sclerosis and Atherosclerosis. Biomolecules. 2019;9(9).

[60] Gossl M, Versari D, Mannheim D, Ritman EL, Lerman LO, Lerman A. Increased spatial vasa vasorum density in the proximal LAD in hypercholesterolemia--implications for vulnerable plaque-development. Atherosclerosis. 2007;192(2):246-52.

[61] Herrmann J, Lerman LO, Rodriguez-Porcel M, Holmes DR, Jr., Richardson DM, Ritman EL, et al. Coronary vasa vasorum neovascularization precedes epicardial endothelial dysfunction in experimental hypercholesterolemia. Cardiovasc Res. 2001;51(4):762-6.

[62] Xu F, Ji J, Li L, Chen R, Hu WC. Adventitial fibroblasts are activated in the early stages of atherosclerosis in the apolipoprotein E knockout mouse. Biochem Biophys Res Commun. 2007;352(3):681-8.

[63] Lin J, Kakkar V, Lu X. Impact of MCP-1 in atherosclerosis. Curr Pharm Des. 2014;20(28):4580-8.

[64] Xu F, Liu Y, Shi L, Liu W, Zhang L, Cai H, et al. NADPH oxidase p47phox siRNA attenuates adventitial fibroblasts proliferation and migration in apoE(−/−) mouse. J Transl Med. 2015;13:38.

[65] Liao DF, Jin ZG, Baas AS, Daum G, Gygi SP, Aebersold R, et al. Purification

and identification of secreted oxidative stress-induced factors from vascular smooth muscle cells. J Biol Chem. 2000;275(1):189-96.

[66] Xu F, Ji J, Li L, Chen R, Hu W. Activation of adventitial fibroblasts contributes to the early development of atherosclerosis: a novel hypothesis that complements the "Response-to-Injury Hypothesis" and the "Inflammation Hypothesis". Med Hypotheses. 2007; 69(4):908-12.

[67] Brokopp CE, Schoenauer R, Richards P, Bauer S, Lohmann C, Emmert MY, et al. Fibroblast activation protein is induced by inflammation and degrades type I collagen in thin-cap fibroatheromata. Eur Heart J. 2011; 32(21):2713-22.

[68] Albanese I, Khan K, Barratt B, Al-Kindi H, Schwertani A. Atherosclerotic Calcification: Wnt Is the Hint. J Am Heart Assoc. 2018;7(4).

[69] Katja Lakota AA, Sasa Cucnik, Jana Brguljan-Hitij, Borut Cegovnik, Barbara Salobir, Rok Accetto, Borut Bozic, Blaz Rozman and Snezna Sodin-Semrl Atherogenesis, Inflammation and Autoimmunity - An Overview. 2012. In: Atherogenesis [Internet]. IntechOpen; [187-202]. Available from: https://www.intechopen.com/books/atherogenesis/atherogenesis-inflammation-and-autoimmunity-an-overview.

[70] Koenig W, Khuseyinova N. Biomarkers of atherosclerotic plaque instability and rupture. Arterioscler Thromb Vasc Biol. 2007;27(1):15-26.

[71] Karanian JW, Peregoy JA, Chiesa OA, Murray TL, Ahn C, Pritchard WF. Efficiency of drug delivery to the coronary arteries in swine is dependent on the route of administration: assessment of luminal, intimal, and adventitial coronary artery and venous delivery methods. J Vasc Interv Radiol. 2010;21(10):1555-64.

[72] Rios CD, Ooboshi H, Piegors D, Davidson BL, Heistad DD. Adenovirus-mediated gene transfer to normal and atherosclerotic arteries. A novel approach. Arterioscler Thromb Vasc Biol. 1995;15(12):2241-5.

[73] Dourron HM, Jacobson GM, Park JL, Liu J, Reddy DJ, Scheel ML, et al. Perivascular gene transfer of NADPH oxidase inhibitor suppresses angioplasty-induced neointimal proliferation of rat carotid artery. Am J Physiol Heart Circ Physiol. 2005;288(2): H946-53.

[74] Stein S, Weber J, Nusser-Stein S, Pahla J, Zhang HE, Mohammed SA, et al. Deletion of fibroblast activation protein provides atheroprotection. Cardiovasc Res. 2021;117(4): 1060-9.

[75] Berry JM, Le V, Rotter D, Battiprolu PK, Grinsfelder B, Tannous P, et al. Reversibility of adverse, calcineurin-dependent cardiac remodeling. Circ Res. 2011;109(4): 407-17.

[76] Patel R, Nagueh SF, Tsybouleva N, Abdellatif M, Lutucuta S, Kopelen HA, et al. Simvastatin induces regression of cardiac hypertrophy and fibrosis and improves cardiac function in a transgenic rabbit model of human hypertrophic cardiomyopathy. Circulation. 2001;104(3):317-24.

[77] Christen T, Verin V, Bochaton-Piallat M, Popowski Y, Ramaekers F, Debruyne P, et al. Mechanisms of neointima formation and remodeling in the porcine coronary artery. Circulation. 2001;103(6):882-8.

[78] Evrard SM, Lecce L, Michelis KC, Nomura-Kitabayashi A, Pandey G, Purushothaman KR, et al. Endothelial to mesenchymal transition is common in atherosclerotic lesions and is associated with plaque instability. Nat Commun. 2016;7:11853.

[79] Bayes-Genis A, Campbell JH, Carlson PJ, Holmes DR, Jr., Schwartz RS. Macrophages, myofibroblasts and neointimal hyperplasia after coronary artery injury and repair. Atherosclerosis. 2002;163(1):89-98.

[80] Shi-Wen X, Chen Y, Denton CP, Eastwood M, Renzoni EA, Bou-Gharios G, et al. Endothelin-1 promotes myofibroblast induction through the ETA receptor via a rac/phosphoinositide 3-kinase/Akt-dependent pathway and is essential for the enhanced contractile phenotype of fibrotic fibroblasts. Mol Biol Cell. 2004;15(6):2707-19.

[81] Shi Y, O'Brien JE, Fard A, Mannion JD, Wang D, Zalewski A. Adventitial myofibroblasts contribute to neointimal formation in injured porcine coronary arteries. Circulation. 1996;94(7):1655-64.

[82] Siow RC, Mallawaarachchi CM, Weissberg PL. Migration of adventitial myofibroblasts following vascular balloon injury: insights from in vivo gene transfer to rat carotid arteries. Cardiovasc Res. 2003;59(1):212-21.

[83] Kato K, Logsdon NJ, Shin YJ, Palumbo S, Knox A, Irish JD, et al. Impaired Myofibroblast Dedifferentiation Contributes to Nonresolving Fibrosis in Aging. Am J Respir Cell Mol Biol. 2020;62(5):633-44.

[84] Yang X, Chen B, Liu T, Chen X. Reversal of myofibroblast differentiation: a review. Eur J Pharmacol. 2014;734:83-90.

[85] Huang S, Wettlaufer SH, Hogaboam C, Aronoff DM, Peters-Golden M. Prostaglandin E(2) inhibits collagen expression and proliferation in patient-derived normal lung fibroblasts via E prostanoid 2 receptor and cAMP signaling. Am J Physiol Lung Cell Mol Physiol. 2007;292(2):L405-13.

[86] Garrison G, Huang SK, Okunishi K, Scott JP, Kumar Penke LR, Scruggs AM, et al. Reversal of myofibroblast differentiation by prostaglandin E(2). Am J Respir Cell Mol Biol. 2013;48(5):550-8.

[87] Artaud-Macari E, Goven D, Brayer S, Hamimi A, Besnard V, Marchal-Somme J, et al. Nuclear factor erythroid 2-related factor 2 nuclear translocation induces myofibroblastic dedifferentiation in idiopathic pulmonary fibrosis. Antioxid Redox Signal. 2013;18(1):66-79.

[88] Maltseva O, Folger P, Zekaria D, Petridou S, Masur SK. Fibroblast growth factor reversal of the corneal myofibroblast phenotype. Invest Ophthalmol Vis Sci. 2001;42(11):2490-5.

[89] Mindur JE, Swirski FK. Growth Factors as Immunotherapeutic Targets in Cardiovascular Disease. Arterioscler Thromb Vasc Biol. 2019;39(7):1275-87.

[90] Itoh N, Ornitz DM. Fibroblast growth factors: from molecular evolution to roles in development, metabolism and disease. J Biochem. 2011;149(2):121-30.

[91] Majesky MW, Horita H, Ostriker A, Lu S, Regan JN, Bagchi A, et al. Differentiated Smooth Muscle Cells Generate a Subpopulation of Resident Vascular Progenitor Cells in the Adventitia Regulated by Klf4. Circ Res. 2017;120(2):296-311.

[92] Hu Y, Zhang Z, Torsney E, Afzal AR, Davison F, Metzler B, et al. Abundant progenitor cells in the adventitia contribute to atherosclerosis of vein grafts in ApoE-deficient mice. J Clin Invest. 2004;113(9):1258-65.

[93] Soundararajan M, Kannan S. Fibroblasts and mesenchymal stem cells:

Two sides of the same coin? J Cell Physiol. 2018;233(12):9099-109.

[94] Ichim TE, O'Heeron P, Kesari S. Fibroblasts as a practical alternative to mesenchymal stem cells. J Transl Med. 2018;16(1):212.

[95] Yu B, Chen Q, Le Bras A, Zhang L, Xu Q. Vascular Stem/Progenitor Cell Migration and Differentiation in Atherosclerosis. Antioxid Redox Signal. 2018;29(2):219-35.

[96] Tang J, Wang H, Huang X, Li F, Zhu H, Li Y, et al. Arterial Sca1(+) Vascular Stem Cells Generate De Novo Smooth Muscle for Artery Repair and Regeneration. Cell Stem Cell. 2020;26(1):81-96 e4.

[97] Wirka RC, Wagh D, Paik DT, Pjanic M, Nguyen T, Miller CL, et al. Atheroprotective roles of smooth muscle cell phenotypic modulation and the TCF21 disease gene as revealed by single-cell analysis. Nat Med. 2019;25(8):1280-9.

[98] Chen PY, Qin L, Baeyens N, Li G, Afolabi T, Budatha M, et al. Endothelial-to-mesenchymal transition drives atherosclerosis progression. J Clin Invest. 2015;125(12):4514-28.

Chapter 4

Heterogeneity of Fibroblasts in Healthy and Diseased Kidneys

Takahisa Yoshikawa, Yuki Sato and Motoko Yanagita

Abstract

Chronic kidney disease (CKD) is a worldwide health problem affecting 9.1% of the world's population. The treatments to prevent the progression of CKD remain limited, however. Resident fibroblasts in the kidneys play crucial roles in the pathological conditions commonly recognized in CKD, such as renal fibrosis, renal anemia, and peritubular capillary loss. Fibroblasts in the kidney provide structural backbone by producing extracellular matrix proteins and produce erythropoietin for normal hematopoiesis under physiological conditions. In the diseased condition, however, fibroblasts differentiate into myofibroblasts that produce excessive extracellular matrix proteins at the cost of the inherent erythropoietin-producing abilities, resulting in renal fibrosis and renal anemia. Pericytes, which are mesenchymal cells that enwrap peritubular capillaries and highly overlap with resident fibroblasts, detach from peritubular capillary walls in response to kidney injury, resulting in peritubular capillary loss and tissue hypoxia. Several reports have demonstrated the beneficial roles of fibroblasts in the regeneration of renal tubules Renal fibroblasts also have the potential to differentiate into a proinflammatory state, producing various cytokines and chemokines and prolonging inflammation by forming tertiary lymphoid tissues, functional lymphoid aggregates, in some pathological conditions. In this article, we describe the heterogenous functions of renal fibroblasts under healthy and diseased conditions.

Keywords: chronic kidney disease, erythropoietin, renal anemia, fibrosis, myofibroblast, tertiary lymphoid tissue

1. Introduction

Chronic kidney disease (CKD) is a worldwide public health problem. In 2017, the prevalence of CKD was estimated to be 9.1% in the world's population, and has increased by 29.3% from 1990 to 2017 [1]. The prevalence of CKD in elderly individuals over 65 years old is especially high and is predicted to increase further as a result of the increasingly aged society [2]. CKD is a risk factor for end-stage renal disease (ESRD) and is also recognized as an independent risk factor for cardiovascular diseases and their associated mortality [3]. Patients with ESRD need renal replacement therapies such as dialysis and renal transplantation to survive. The cost of these therapies is enormous and the financial burden is a critical problem for patients and society [4]. Nevertheless, treatment to prevent the progression of CKD and the occurrence of CKD-associated complications remain limited.

IntechOpen

Fibroblasts are distributed in various organs throughout the body and contribute to both homeostasis and disease. In the kidney, resident fibroblasts play crucial roles in both health and disease, and their phenotypes are heterogenous and plastic [5]. Under physiological conditions, renal fibroblasts provide structural support for the entire kidney architecture and produce erythropoietin (EPO). In contrast, in diseased kidneys, fibroblasts lose these physiological functions and transdifferentiate into myofibroblasts. These phenotypic changes result in fibrosis, renal anemia, and peritubular capillary loss, all of which are common pathological conditions of CKD, irrespective of the etiology [6]. Renal fibroblasts also act as inflammatory cells and produce proinflammatory cytokines and chemokines under some pathological conditions [5, 7]. In aged injured kidneys, fibroblasts play a crucial role in prolonging inflammation by inducing tertiary lymphoid tissue (TLT) formation [8]. These features highlight the importance of understanding the behavior of fibroblasts in the kidney in order to identify efficient therapeutic strategies to prevent CKD progression. In this article, we describe the current understanding of the heterogeneous functions of fibroblasts in healthy and diseased kidneys.

2. Fibroblasts in the kidney

2.1 Characteristics and functions of resident fibroblasts in kidneys

Renal resident fibroblasts are spindle-shaped cells that exist in the interstitial space, which is defined as the area between nephrons. Nephrons are functional units of the kidney and are composed of glomerular and tubular cells. Fibroblasts provide the structural backbone of the kidney by producing extracellular matrix (ECM) proteins and interact with surrounding cells to maintain the homeostatic state in healthy kidneys. Identification of resident fibroblasts is performed based on their location, shape, and positive expressions of several fibroblast markers such as CD73 and PDGFRβ [9]. As these markers are neither homogeneously positive nor specific for resident fibroblasts, confirming the negative expression of other cell-lineage markers such as CD45, a hematopoietic cell marker, is also necessary to identify renal resident fibroblasts.

In addition to the role of structural cells, fibroblasts have unique organ-specific functions. In the kidney, small subset of the renal resident fibroblasts residing in the corticomedullary area produces Epo, a hormone essential for erythropoiesis in response to hypoxia [10]. Although there are few Epo-producing cells and they exist only in the deep cortex in the physiological state, under severe hypoxic conditions such as severe anemia, the number of Epo-producing cells increases and they can be detected in the cortical area [11]. The increase in the number of Epo-producing cells under hypoxic conditions is likely due to the increase in the number of the cells that have acquired Epo-producing ability but not to cellular proliferation, because Epo production is activated in anemic mice under administration of a cell cycle inhibitor or γ-ray irradiation [10]. Interestingly, while other growth factors for hematopoietic cells (such as granulocyte colony-stimulating factor) are produced in bone marrow, where hematopoietic cells are generated and the growth factors are required, EPO is produced from the kidney. One possible explanation for this is that kidneys are physiologically hypoxic compared with other organs, which allows them to be more sensitive to small changes in oxygen delivery than other organs and is advantageous to the production of EPO in response to hypoxia [12]. Another explanation is that kidneys function as a "critmeter," with the ability to set hematocrit within the normal range by regulating plasma volume and the red blood cell mass in a common site [13].

2.2 Origin and heterogeneity of fibroblasts in the kidney

In 1974, Le Douarin et al. reported that, in transplantation experiments of quail neural tubes to chicks, quail neural crest–derived cells were identified in the renal interstitial space [14]. Consistently, we found that fibroblasts in neonate kidneys express p75 neurotrophin receptor (p75NTR), a neural crest marker [15]. Moreover, Epo-producing cells express neuronal markers such as microtubule-associated protein 2 and neurofilament light polypeptide [10]. Based on these previous findings, we conducted a lineage tracing study using *myelin protein zero (P0)-Cre* mice, which label neural crest–derived cells, and found that resident fibroblasts in the cortex and corticomedullary area are lineage-labeled with *P0-Cre* [15]. We also demonstrated that, in embryonic kidneys, *P0-Cre* lineage–labeled cells appeared in the interstitial space along the outer capsule and ureter from E13.5 and more than 99% of the resident fibroblasts in the cortex and outer medulla were labeled with *P0-Cre* in adult kidneys. Consistently, Epo-producing fibroblasts were also labeled with *P0-Cre* in the experiment using *P0-Cre:R26R:EPO-GFP* mice [15]. In contrast, renal fibroblasts in the medulla are not labeled with *P0-Cre*. Wnt4 expression is identified in the medullary stromal mesenchyme in embryotic kidneys and reactivated in medullary fibroblasts after renal injury [16, 17]. These findings suggest the regional heterogeneity of fibroblasts and their origin in the adult kidney. The functional heterogeneity of PDGFRβ^+ Epo-producing cells was also reported. Precise histological analysis showed that different subpopulations of fibroblasts produce Epo responding to different stimuli [18].

2.3 Pericytes in kidneys

Pericytes are mesenchyme-derived cells that enwrap capillaries with their processes embedded in the vascular basement membrane. Resident fibroblasts and pericytes share several characteristics, including their interstitial location and cell surface markers such as CD73 and PDGFRβ, and, as such, these two types of cells are often confused. Pericytes support the capillary structure and regulate vascular tone with their contraction force [19]. Moreover, they interact with endothelial cells to maintain capillary homeostasis [6]. Humphreys et al. reported that the origins of pericytes in the kidneys were FoxD1-expressing cells in an experiment using *FoxD1-Cre* mice [20]. On the other hand, it was reported that *P0-Cre* lineage–labeled cells in E13.5 embryonic kidneys transiently expressed FoxD1 [15]. Based on these findings, it is assumed that resident fibroblasts and pericytes are highly overlapped populations in the kidneys.

3. Renal fibrosis as a hallmark of CKD

Renal fibrosis is a common pathological condition of CKD, irrespective of the etiology. It is defined as excessive accumulation of ECM such as collagen and fibronectin in the interstitial space and is recognized as a predictive indicator of renal prognosis [21]. Previous studies have shown that dysfunction of the renal fibroblasts can induce several pathological conditions associated with CKD, such as renal fibrosis, renal anemia, and peritubular capillary loss. Against this background, renal fibroblasts have been focused on as hopeful therapeutic targets for CKD and its complications.

3.1 Myofibroblasts in kidneys and their origin

Myofibroblasts are recognized as the main contributor to fibrosis in multiple organs. They are characterized by dense endoplasmic reticulum and contractile microfilament bundles [22]. Their most prominent feature is the expression of α-smooth muscle actin (α-SMA) that forms myofilament bundles and promotes their high contractility [23]. Although myofibroblasts are almost undetectable in healthy kidneys, they expand dramatically in diseased kidneys and drive fibrosis by producing a large amount of ECM proteins and through their own proliferation. The origin of myofibroblasts has been discussed for decades, and several genetic lineage tracing studies recently revealed that resident fibroblasts and pericytes are the main sources for myofibroblasts [9]. We reported that *P0-Cre* lineage–labeled cells, which were progenitors of resident fibroblasts (as mentioned above), could differentiate into myofibroblasts in several kidney injury models [15]. Humphreys et al. reported that *FoxD1-Cre* lineage–labeled pericytes are the main sources for myofibroblasts [20]. These studies demonstrated that most myofibroblasts are derived from these renal fibroblasts and pericytes. Although several studies have reported other types of cells as progenitor cells for myofibroblasts, such as epithelial cells, endothelial cells, and hematopoietic cells, recent lineage tracing experiments demonstrated that tubular epithelial cells do not become myofibroblasts *in vivo* [20, 24, 25]. The endothelial-to-mesenchymal transition, in which endothelial cells transdifferentiate into myofibroblasts, was also reported to contribute less to myofibroblast pools than resident fibroblasts [24]. Additionally, Kramman et al. used single-cell RNA sequencing (scRNA-seq) and parabiosis techniques to demonstrate the limited contribution of circulating monocytes to myofibroblast pools with very few matrix genes expression in murine fibrotic kidneys [25].

Notably, although genetic lineage tracing is not feasible in humans, a recent study utilizing scRNA-seq of human kidney samples supports the notion that these findings in mice appear to be conserved in humans. Kuppe et al. conducted scRNA-seq on human kidneys in patients with CKD and demonstrated that Notch3$^+$ pericytes and Meg3$^+$ fibroblasts were the main sources for highly ECM-producing myofibroblasts using pseudo-time trajectory analysis and diffusion map analysis [26]. These studies support the idea that most renal myofibroblasts derive from renal resident fibroblasts or pericytes.

3.2 Progenitor of myofibroblasts; Gli1$^+$ fibroblasts in the perivascular niche

Mesenchymal stem cells (MSCs) are defined as cells with self-renewal and clonogenic capacity. Gli1$^+$ fibroblasts are MSC-like cells that reside in both the pericyte niche and the adventitia of larger vessels across multiple organs, including the kidney, and exhibit trilineage differentiation potential *in vitro* [27, 28]. A fate tracing study utilizing *Gli1-CreERt2:tdTomato* reporter mice revealed that, although Gli1$^+$ fibroblasts represented only 0.2% of the PDGFRβ$^+$ renal fibroblast population in healthy kidneys, after renal injury, they proliferated dramatically, mainly in the medulla and inner cortex, and differentiated into αSMA$^+$ myofibroblasts. Additionally, using *Gli1-CreERt2:iDTR* (inducible diphtheria toxin receptor) mice, the ablation of Gli1$^+$ cells by diphtheria toxin (DT) administration dramatically reduced renal fibrosis by approximately 50% after unilateral ureteral obstruction (UUO), which is an *in vivo* experimental model of renal fibrosis. These data suggested that Gli1$^+$ fibroblasts predominantly proliferated and contributed to renal fibrosis, suggesting the heterogeneity of the potential to transdifferentiate into myofibroblasts among PDGFRβ$^+$ fibroblasts in the kidney.

3.3 The roles of proximal tubule injury in CKD progression

Acute kidney injury (AKI) is a highly prevalent disorder and is one of the risk factors for the progression of CKD [29]. The underlying molecular mechanisms for CKD transition after AKI have been investigated for decades. The proximal tubules are the most vulnerable segment in the nephron, and are assumed to trigger the AKI to CKD progression. To investigate whether injured proximal tubules can trigger renal fibrosis, we selectively damaged proximal tubules by DT administration in *Ndrg1-CreERt2:iDTR* mice, in which DTR is specifically expressed on proximal tubules in the kidneys [30]. Low-dose single DT administration caused mild proximal tubule injury and reversible fibrosis whereas high-dose single DT or repeated low-dose DT administration caused sustained renal fibrosis. This study showed that injury of the proximal tubules is sufficient to cause several features of CKD, and that the frequency and severity of proximal tubule injury are associated with the degree of AKI to CKD progression. As an explanation for the association between proximal tubule injury and CKD, tubulointerstitial interactions in injured kidneys have been reported to contribute to renal fibrosis [31]. Yang et al. demonstrated that, in a multiple profibrotic AKI model, injured proximal tubules underwent cell cycle arrest in G2/M and acquired the profibrotic secretory phenotype by upregulating profibrotic cytokine production, such as transforming growth factor β-1 (TGFβ-1) and connective tissue growth factor [32]. Additionally, the administration of a p53 inhibitor, a therapy employed for bypassing G2/M arrest, attenuated renal fibrosis in a renal ischemic reperfusion injury model. Injured proximal tubules have been reported to secrete several other profibrotic ligands expressed during renal development. The Wnt family plays a crucial role in kidney development, and many Wnt family genes are upregulated in fibrotic kidney models [33]. Zhou et al. demonstrated that the selective ablation of Wntless, a cargo receptor necessary for Wnt secretion, in renal tubular epithelial cells but not in interstitial fibroblasts attenuated renal fibrosis in a UUO model, suggesting that the Wnt family secreted by renal tubules contributed to renal fibrosis. Moreover, Maarouf et al. showed that Wnt1 expression genetically induced in proximal tubules was sufficient for renal fibrogenesis by inducing interstitial myofibroblast activation and proliferation [34]. According to these reports, one of the mechanisms of the AKI to CKD transition is that ligands secreted from injured renal tubules contribute to renal fibrogenesis by activating myofibroblasts.

4. Two common CKD complications, renal anemia and peritubular capillary loss, are also caused by dysfunction of renal fibroblasts/pericytes

Renal anemia is a common complication that affects the majority of patients with CKD [35]. The cause of renal anemia is the relative deficiency of EPO. Several recent studies have shown that dysfunction of renal fibroblasts contribute to this complication. EPO production is stimulated by hypoxia and regulated by hypoxia-inducible factors (HIFs). In normoxic conditions, HIFs are hydroxylated by HIF-prolyl hydroxylase domain–containing proteins (PHDs), and hydroxylated HIFs are degraded by the ubiquitin-proteasome system [36, 37]. In hypoxic conditions, the hydroxylation and degradation of HIFs is inhibited, resulting in the transcriptional activation of HIF-inducible genes, including *EPO*. In renal fibrosis models, the Epo-producing fibroblasts transdifferentiate into myofibroblasts in response to kidney injury and decrease the capacity to produce Epo at the same time [11, 15, 38]. Souma et al. demonstrated that activation of HIFs by the genetic inactivation of PHDs in Epo-producing cells restored Epo production in Epo-producing cell–derived myofibroblasts in a renal fibrosis model [39]. Additionally, severe anemia or the administration of selective estrogen receptor modulators, the neuroprotective agents, neurotrophin, and the renoprotective agent, hepatocyte growth factor, restored the ability to produce Epo in myofibroblasts [15]. These results demonstrated that the ability to produce Epo in myofibroblasts has plasticity and can be restored by therapeutic interventions. As for the mechanism of the decrease of Epo production in myofibroblasts, Souma et al. showed that NFκB signaling repressed Epo production in fibroblasts in UUO models. Moreover, *Epo-Cre:R26-IKK2ca/+* mice, in which NFκB signals in Epo-producing cells were selectively activated, showed that 20% of Epo-producing cells were positive for α-SMA, suggesting that NFκB signaling also contributed to the transition of EPO-producing fibroblasts into myofibroblasts [11]. Another possible mechanism for the repression of Epo production in myofibroblasts is that hypermethylation in the *Epo* promotor, which is induced by TGFβ-1 stimulation, inhibits *Epo* expression in myofibroblasts in the fibrotic kidney [38]. Fuchs et al. also showed that Epo production in renal fibroblasts was suppressed by TGFβ signaling in renal fibrosis models, utilizing *PDGFRβ-Cre:TGFβ-R2*$^{fl/fl}$ mice, and hypothesized that it occurred before the phenotypic shift of fibroblasts to myofibroblasts because the frequency of α-SMA$^+$ myofibroblasts did not differ between the knockout mice and control mice [40].

Although the administration of erythropoiesis-stimulating agents (ESAs) is a currently well-established and effective clinical treatment, it might be associated with several adverse effects, such as hypertension and thrombotic complications [41]. To avoid safety concerns associated with ESAs, PHD inhibitors, which upregulate EPO production via the stabilization of HIFs, have been developed and used for the treatment of renal anemia [36, 42–45].

Another common pathological feature of CKD is the loss of peritubular capillaries [46]. Renal pericytes enwrap peritubular capillaries and support them structurally. In response to injury, pericytes detach from capillaries and their processes, which form networks surrounding the capillaries, start to direct from their associated capillaries to the adjacent tubules, concomitant with transdifferentiation into myofibroblasts [39]. This pathological change makes peritubular capillaries unstable and causes capillary rarefaction and loss [47]. Reduced peritubular capillary blood supply can cause chronic hypoxia in renal parenchymal cells such as tubules and stromal cells. Hypoxia aggravates renal fibrosis by stimulating fibroblasts and altering their gene expressions associated with ECM metabolism [48]. For example, hypoxia upregulated collagen type 1 and the tissue inhibitor of metalloproteinase-1 expression and also downregulated matrix metalloproteinase-1 *in vitro*, which led to the accumulation of ECM proteins. Excessive fibrosis also reduces the efficiency of oxygen diffusion due to the expanded distance between capillaries and tubules and induces renal damage, which can drive further CKD progression. Recently, a sodium-glucose cotransporter 2 (SGLT2) inhibitor, which prevents glucose reabsorption by SGLT2 in proximal tubules, was reported to prevent tissue hypoxia and renal fibrosis in an ischemic reperfusion injury (IRI) model by ameliorating renal capillary rarefaction and the detachment of pericytes from endothelial cells with the promotion of vascular endothelial growth factor-A expression in proximal tubular cells [49]. Additionally, SGLT2 inhibitor treatment was reported to increase hematocrit concomitantly with the elevation of serum EPO concentrations in patients with type 2 diabetes mellitus [50, 51]. On the basis of these reports, SGLT2 inhibitors are expected to play a beneficial role in the restoration of the physiological functions of fibroblasts.

5. Beneficial function of myofibroblasts in kidneys

Contrary to the long-held assumption that fibrosis is detrimental to the host, recent evidence suggests that fibrosis also has host-protective roles in some cases. To investigate the role of fibroblasts during the early phase of kidney injury, we utilized *P0-Cre:iDTR* mice [52], which allow us to induce resident fibroblast-specific dysfunction at the desired time point by DT administration. Utilizing this system, we found that the dysfunction of resident fibroblasts in the acute phase of injury impaired tubular regeneration. During the transition from fibroblasts to myofibroblasts, fibroblasts upregulate the expression of retinaldehyde dehydrogenase 2 (RALDH2), a rate-limiting enzyme in retinoic acid (RA) synthesis. Given that RAs are essential for kidney development, RAs derived from myofibroblasts might promote tubule regeneration. Retinoic acid receptor (RAR) γ and the downstream molecules such as αB-crystallin were expressed in proximal tubules in injured kidneys, and the administration of an RAR inverse agonist to the proximal tubule cell line attenuated proliferation *in vitro*. Another example of the beneficial role of fibroblasts during injury was shown by the experiment utilizing the intravital imaging method [53]. Schiessl et al. demonstrated that, in response to laser-induced tubular cell injury, PDGFRβ$^+$ interstitial cells migrated towards tubular injury sites and enclosed the injured tubules. Additionally, PDGFRβ inhibitors compromised the recruitment of the interstitial cells and tubule regeneration. These results suggest that fibroblasts have the potential to promote tubule regeneration, at least in the acute phase of kidney injury, via PDGFRβ signaling.

6. Renal fibroblasts associated with inflammation

Although myofibroblasts are established as the primary effector cells driving fibrosis, several recent studies have demonstrated that resident fibroblasts in the kidney also have a proinflammatory phenotype. Souma et al. reported that Epo-producing fibroblast–derived myofibroblasts upregulated the expression of the target genes of NFκB such as *Il6* and *Ccl2* in an UUO model [11]. Leaf et al. reported that renal pericytes could work as innate immune cells and respond to damage-associated molecular patterns (DAMPs) sensitively in the acute phase of renal injury [54]. In response to the stimulation with DAMPs, renal pericytes activated NLRP3 inflammasome and secreted IL-1β and IL-18 in a TLR2/TLR4 and Myd88-dependent manner and aggravated renal fibrosis in the IRI model. *In vitro*, Myd88 knockout pericytes and Tlr2/Tlr4 double knockout pericytes also reduced their ability to migrate and the expression of the genes associated with fibrosis in response to TGF-β or DAMPs. These results suggested that both the inflammatory and fibrogenic properties of pericytes were dependent on Myd88, TLR2, and TLR4. Further studies are necessary to elucidate the significance of proinflammatory fibroblasts in renal injury and CKD progression.

It is of note that an anti-inflammatory role of fibroblasts and pericytes was also reported. Using *FoxD1-Cre:CD73*$^{fl/fl}$ mice, Perry et al. demonstrated that CD73, an enzyme converting AMP to adenosine on fibroblasts and pericytes, was necessary to suppress inflammation and attenuate renal fibrosis after kidney injury [55]. Additionally, the absence of CD73 on the fibroblasts was associated with an increase in α-SMA expression *in vitro*. The authors hypothesized that the adenosine locally generated by CD73 on fibroblasts and pericytes might act on adenosine receptors in an autocrine and paracrine manner and attenuate macrophage infiltration and profibrotic properties. Importantly, renal fibroblasts can act as modulators of inflammation and contribute to normal tissue repair by interacting with the surrounding cells.

7. Age-dependent phenotype of fibroblasts: tertiary lymphoid tissue: associated fibroblasts

7.1 Tertiary lymphoid tissue formation in aged injured kidneys

An epidemiological study showed that elderly patients with AKI had an increased risk for CKD progression [56]. The mechanism for the maladaptive repair after AKI in the elderly remains unknown. To identify the mechanism, we compared the renal response to injury between young and aged mice. As in humans, while young kidney repaired itself after injury, aged kidney exhibited sustained tubular injury and fibrosis [8]. Unexpectedly, we found multiple TLTs in aged kidneys but not young kidneys in the chronic phase after kidney injury. TLT is an ectopic lymphoid tissue that develops at the site of chronic inflammation. TLTs are mainly composed of lymphocytes that are structurally and functionally supported by unique phenotypic fibroblasts inside TLTs (**Figure 1**). Unlike simple infiltration of the inflammatory cells, TLTs can promote lymphocyte proliferation and differentiation, resulting in the generation of antibody-secreting plasma cells, as recognized in secondary lymphoid organs [57]. Importantly, although TLTs are identified in various disease conditions, such as autoimmune diseases, infections, and cancers, TLTs can play beneficial or pathological roles in a context-dependent manner [58]. For example, in chronic inflammatory or autoimmune diseases, TLTs contribute to disease persistence and have detrimental effects on the host [59]. In contrast, during infections, TLTs are assumed to play beneficial roles to eliminate pathogens by promoting immune responses [60]. The role of TLTs in aged injured kidneys remains unclear, and will be discussed in the next section.

7.2 Characteristics and origin of fibroblasts inside tertiary lymphoid tissues

Fibroblasts inside TLTs exhibit unique characteristics that are distinct from those outside TLTs, such as the strong expression of p75NTR (**Figure 1**) [8]. After kidney injury, resident fibroblasts acquire the ability to produce RAs by upregulating RALDH2, which is assumed to promote the transition of the adjacent fibroblasts into $p75NTR^+$ TLT-associated fibroblasts. Some of the $p75NTR^+$ TLT-associated fibroblasts acquire abilities to secrete homeostatic chemokines such as CCL19 and CXCL13, which are the driving force for recruiting lymphocytes and promoting TLT

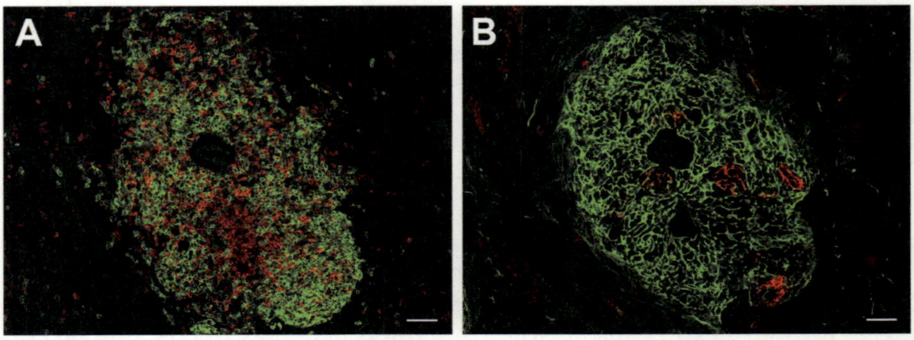

Figure 1.
Tertiary lymphoid tissues in aged murine kidney 45 days after ischemic reperfusion injury. (A) Immuno fluorescence staining of B220 (green) and CD3ε (red). Tertiary lymphoid tissues (TLTs) are mainly composed of $B220^+$ B cells and $CD3ε^+$ T cells. (B) Immunofluorescence staining of p75NTR (green) and CD21 (red). Fibroblasts inside TLTs express p75 neurotrophin receptor (p75NTR). In mature TLTs, some of the fibroblasts differentiate into $p75NTR^-/CD21^+$ follicular dendritic cells. Scale bar: 50 μm.

formation. Inside of more mature TLTs, $CD21^+/p75NTR^-$ follicular dendritic cells (FDCs) appear as part of stromal cells (**Figure 1**). FDCs are stromal cells residing in the B cell follicles of secondary lymphoid organs; they drive germinal center reactions [61]. These TLT-associated fibroblasts in the kidneys are *P0-Cre* lineage–labeled cells, suggesting that renal resident fibroblasts can differentiate into these various types of fibroblasts [8].

7.3 Clinical significance of tertiary lymphoid tissues in CKD and the elderly

Several studies have reported that TLTs are induced in various kidney diseases [62–65]. Additionally, we reported that TLTs developed not only in murine kidneys but also in human kidneys in an age-dependent manner [8]. In the analysis on kidneys from nephrectomy cases for renal cell carcinoma and autopsy, excluding pyelonephritis, glomerulonephritis, autoimmune kidney diseases, and hematological malignancies, TLTs were identified only in the elderly over 60 years old. The components of human TLTs are quite similar to those of murine TLTs. To evaluate TLTs objectively, we classified renal TLTs into three stages based on the immunostaining patterns as follows [66]. TLTs not containing $CD21^+$ FDCs or a germinal center response, dense $Ki67^+$ proliferative B cell clusters, were defined as stage 1. TLTs containing $CD21^+$ FDCs but no germinal center response were defined as stage 2. TLTs containing both $CD21^+$ FDCs and a germinal center response were defined as stage 3. In this classification, the severity of the TLT stages and the area of TLTs were related with the severity of ischemic injury in murine renal IRI models. In humans, more and higher-stage TLTs were identified in the kidneys of patients with CKD than without CKD among elderly patients 60 years or older in the analysis using kidneys from nephrectomy cases due to renal cell carcinoma [66]. These data demonstrated that the developmental stage of TLTs was associated with the severity of kidney injury, thereby indicating that TLTs have potential as a marker of severity of renal injury.

7.4 Potential of tertiary lymphoid tissues as therapeutic targets for CKD

Although TLTs are assumed to be associated with the severity of renal injury, it has been challenging to determine whether renal TLTs are pathogenic and if they directly affect renal function. We reported that, in unilateral renal IRI models of aged mice, the administration of GK1.5, anti-CD4 monoclonal antibody, diminished TLT formation and inflammatory marker expressions and improved renal fibrosis [8]. This result suggests that renal TLTs could be pathogenic and the therapies targeting renal TLTs thus have the potential to improve renal function in patients with CKD. As this intervention is not specific to TLTs and affects systemic immune systems, however, a more specific therapy for TLTs is necessary to determine whether TLTs in aged injured kidneys are detrimental or not.

8. Conclusion

Resident fibroblasts in the kidney are essential components to maintain homeostasis under physiological conditions. In CKD, dysfunction of renal fibroblasts causes the main pathological conditions of renal fibrosis, renal anemia, and peritubular capillary loss. Importantly, renal fibroblasts are heterogeneous and have the potential to change their phenotypes depending on the local microenvironment (**Figure 2**) [5]. Although myofibroblasts mainly contribute to renal fibrosis and deteriorate renal function by producing excessive ECM, they can also

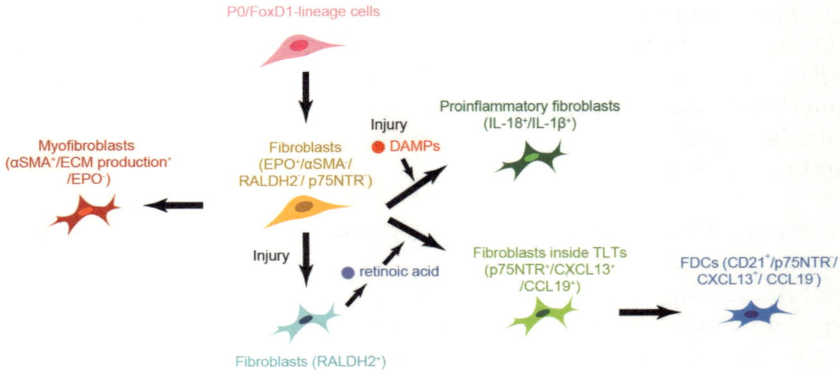

Figure 2.
Heterogeneity of fibroblasts in kidneys. Renal fibroblasts derive from P0- or FoxD1-Cre lineage–labeled cells. Renal fibroblasts change their phenotypes depending on the local microenvironment. Myofibroblasts have the potential to produce excessive extracellular matrix proteins at the cost of EPO production. In response to released DAMPs after injury, fibroblasts can differentiate into proinflammatory fibroblasts that produce IL-18 and IL-1β. In contrast, in aged kidneys, retinoic acids produced by activated fibroblasts after injury induce the differentiation of adjacent fibroblasts into p75NTR⁺ fibroblasts, which produce homeostatic chemokines such as CXCL13 and CCL19, resulting in tertiary lymphoid tissue (TLT) formation. These chemokine-producing fibroblasts can further differentiate into CD21⁺/p75NTR⁻ FDCs in mature TLTs.

have host-protective roles in the early phase of kidney injury. Renal fibroblasts can differentiate into proinflammatory fibroblasts that secrete inflammatory cytokines and chemokines, which can promote TLT formation under several diseased conditions. Fibroblasts or pericytes also have an anti-inflammatory function via CD73 expression. A better understanding of the heterogeneity and roles of renal fibroblasts might lead to the development of a new therapeutic approach for kidney diseases. Recent novel technologies such as scRNA-seq have revealed the heterogeneity of renal fibroblasts that had not previously been identified by conventional technologies [26]. The application of these technologies to various clinical renal diseases is expected to further clarify the heterogeneity of renal fibroblasts, which will result in an enhanced understanding of the pathophysiology of kidney diseases and the development of novel treatments.

Conflict of interest

YS is employed by the TMK Project, which is a collaboration between Kyoto University and Mitsubishi Tanabe Pharma. MY receives research grants from Mitsubishi Tanabe Pharma and Boehringer Ingelheim. TY reports no conflicts of interest.

Appendices and nomenclature

CKD	chronic kidney disease
ESRD	end-stage renal disease
EPO	erythropoietin
TLT	tertiary lymphoid tissue
ECM	extracellular matrix
p75NTR	p75 neurotrophin receptor
P0	myelin protein zero
α-SMA	α-smooth muscle actin

scRNA-seq	single cell RNA-sequencing
MSC	mesenchymal stem cell
iDTR	inducible diphtheria toxin receptor
DT	diphtheria toxin
UUO	unilateral ureteral obstruction
AKI	acute kidney injury
TGFβ-1	transforming growth factor β-1
HIF	hypoxia-inducible factor
PHD	prolyl hydroxylase domain–containing protein
ESA	erythropoiesis-stimulating agent
SGLT2	sodium-glucose cotransporter 2
RALDH2	retinaldehyde dehydrogenase 2
RA	retinoic acid
RAR	retinoic acids receptor
DAMP	damage-associated molecular pattern
FDC	follicular dendritic cell

Author details

Takahisa Yoshikawa[1], Yuki Sato[1,2] and Motoko Yanagita[1,3]*

1 Department of Nephrology, Graduate School of Medicine, Kyoto University, Kyoto, Japan

2 Medical Innovation Center, TMK Project, Graduate School of Medicine, Kyoto University, Kyoto, Japan

3 Institute for the Advanced Study of Human Biology (ASHBi), Kyoto University, Kyoto, Japan

*Address all correspondence to: motoy@kuhp.kyoto-u.ac.jp

References

[1] Bikbov B, Purcell CA, Levey AS, Smith M, Abdoli A, Abebe M, et al. Global, regional, and national burden of chronic kidney disease, 1990-2017: a systematic analysis for the Global Burden of Disease Study 2017. Lancet. 2020;395:709-733. DOI: 10.1016/S0140-6736(20)30045-3

[2] Stevens LA, Li S, Wang C, Huang C, Becker BN, Bomback AS, et al. Prevalence of CKD and Comorbid Illness in Elderly Patients in the United States: Results From the Kidney Early Evaluation Program (KEEP). Am J Kidney Dis. 2010;55:S23–S33. DOI: 10.1053/j.ajkd.2009.09.035 http://dx.doi.org/10.1053/j.ajkd.2009.09.035

[3] Sarnak MJ, Levey AS, Schoolwerth AC, Coresh J, Culleton B, Hamm LL, et al. Kidney Disease as a Risk Factor for Development of Cardiovascular Disease: A Statement From the American Heart Association Councils on Kidney in Cardiovascular Disease, High Blood Pressure Research, Clinical Cardiology, and Epidemiology and Prevention. Circulation. 2003;108:2154-2169. DOI: 10.1161/01.CIR.0000095676.90936.80

[4] Mills KT, Xu Y, Zhang W, Bundy JD, Chen CS, Kelly TN, et al. A systematic analysis of worldwide population-based data on the global burden of chronic kidney disease in 2010. Kidney Int. 2015;88:950-957. DOI: 10.1038/ki.2015.230

[5] Sato Y, Yanagita M. Functional heterogeneity of resident fibroblasts in the kidney. Proc Japan Acad Ser B Phys Biol Sci. 2019;95:468-478. DOI: 10.2183/pjab.95.033

[6] Kramann R, Humphreys BD. Kidney pericytes: Roles in regeneration and fibrosis. Semin Nephrol. 2014;34:374-383. DOI: 10.1016/j.semnephrol.2014.06.004

[7] Sato Y, Yanagita M. Resident fibroblasts in the kidney: A major driver of fibrosis and inflammation. Inflamm Regen. 2017;37:1-7. DOI: 10.1186/s41232-017-0048-3

[8] Sato Y, Mii A, Hamazaki Y, Fujita H, Nakata H, Masuda K, et al. Heterogeneous fibroblasts underlie age-dependent tertiary lymphoid tissues in the kidney. JCI Insight. 2016;1:e87680. DOI: 10.1172/jci.insight.87680

[9] Mack M, Yanagita M. Origin of myofibroblasts and cellular events triggering fibrosis. Kidney Int. 2015;87:297-307. DOI: 10.1038/ki.2014.287

[10] Obara N, Suzuki N, Kim K, Nagasawa T, Imagawa S, Yamamoto M. Repression via the GATA box is essential for tissue-specific erythropoietin gene expression. Blood. 2008;111:5223-5232. DOI: 10.1182/blood-2007-10-115857

[11] Souma T, Yamazaki S, Moriguchi T, Suzuki N, Hirano I, Pan X, et al. Plasticity of renal erythropoietin-producing cells governs fibrosis. J Am Soc Nephrol. 2013;24:1599-1616. DOI: 10.1681/ASN.2013010030

[12] Nangaku M, Eckardt KU. Hypoxia and the HIF system in kidney disease. J Mol Med. 2007;85:1325-1330. DOI: 10.1007/s00109-007-0278-y

[13] Donnelly S. Why is erythropoietin made in the kidney? The kidney functions as a Critmeter. Am J Kidney Dis. 2001;38:415-425. DOI: 10.1053/ajkd.2001.26111

[14] Le Douarin NM, Teillet MAM. Experimental analysis of the migration and differentiation of neuroblasts of the autonomic nervous system and of neurectodermal mesenchymal derivatives, using a biological cell marking technique. Dev Biol.

1974;41:162-184. DOI: 10.1016/0012-1606(74)90291-7

[15] Asada N, Takase M, Nakamura J, Oguchi A, Asada M, Suzuki N, et al. Dysfunction of fibroblasts of extrarenal origin underlies renal fibrosis and renal anemia in mice. J Clin Invest. 2011;121:3981-3990. DOI: 10.1172/JCI57301

[16] Itäranta P, Chi L, Seppänen T, Niku M, Tuukkanen J, Peltoketo H, et al. Wnt-4 signaling is involved in the control of smooth muscle cell fate via Bmp-4 in the medullary stroma of the developing kidney. Dev Biol. 2006;293:473-483. DOI: 10.1016/j.ydbio.2006.02.019

[17] DiRocco DP, Kobayashi A, Taketo MM, McMahon AP, Humphreys BD. Wnt4/β-catenin signaling in medullary kidney myofibroblasts. J Am Soc Nephrol. 2013;24:1399-1412. DOI: 10.1681/ASN.2012050512

[18] Broeker KAE, Fuchs MAA, Schrankl J, Kurt B, Nolan KA, Wenger RH, et al. Different subpopulations of kidney interstitial cells produce erythropoietin and factors supporting tissue oxygenation in response to hypoxia in vivo. Kidney Int. 2020;98:918-931. DOI: 10.1016/j.kint.2020.04.040

[19] Shaw I, Rider S, Mullins J, Hughes J, Péault B. Pericytes in the renal vasculature: Roles in health and disease. Nat Rev Nephrol. 2018;14:521-534. DOI: 10.1038/s41581-018-0032-4

[20] Humphreys BD, Lin SL, Kobayashi A, Hudson TE, Nowlin BT, Bonventre J V., et al. Fate tracing reveals the pericyte and not epithelial origin of myofibroblasts in kidney fibrosis. Am J Pathol. 2010;176:85-97. DOI: 10.2353/ajpath.2010.090517

[21] Nath KA. Tubulointerstitial Changes as a Major Determinant in the Progression of Renal Damage. Am J Kidney Dis. 1992;20:1-17. DOI: 10.1016/S0272-6386(12)80312-X

[22] Klingberg F, Hinz B, White ES. The myofibroblast matrix: Implications for tissue repair andfibrosis. J Pathol. 2013;229:298-309. DOI: 10.1002/path.4104

[23] Kramann R, Dirocco DP, Humphreys BD. Understanding the origin, activation and regulation of matrix-producing myofibroblasts for treatment of fibrotic disease. J Pathol. 2013;231:273-289. DOI: 10.1002/path.4253

[24] Lebleu VS, Taduri G, O'Connell J, Teng Y, Cooke VG, Woda C, et al. Origin and function of myofibroblasts in kidney fibrosis. Nat Med. 2013;19:1047-1053. DOI: 10.1038/nm.3218

[25] Kramann R, Machado F, Wu H, Kusaba T, Hoeft K, Schneider RK, et al. Parabiosis and single-cell RNA sequencing reveal a limited contribution of monocytes to myofibroblasts in kidney fibrosis. JCI insight. 2018;3:e99561. DOI: 10.1172/jci.insight.99561

[26] Kuppe C, Ibrahim MM, Kranz J, Zhang X, Ziegler S, Perales-Patón J, et al. Decoding myofibroblast origins in human kidney fibrosis. Nature. 2021;589:281-286. DOI: 10.1038/s41586-020-2941-1

[27] Kramann R, Schneider RK, Dirocco DP, Machado F, Fleig S, Bondzie PA, et al. Perivascular Gli1+ progenitors are key contributors to injury-induced organ fibrosis. Cell Stem Cell. 2015;16:51-66. DOI: 10.1016/j.stem.2014.11.004

[28] Kramann R, Wongboonsin J, Chang-Panesso M, Machado FG, Humphreys BD. Gli1+ pericyte loss induces capillary rarefaction and proximal tubular injury. J Am Soc

Nephrol. 2017;28:776-784. DOI: 10.1681/ASN.2016030297

[29] Lewington AJP, Cerdá J, Mehta RL. Raising awareness of acute kidney injury: A global perspective of a silent killer. Kidney Int. 2013;84:457-467. 10.1038/ki.2013.153

[30] Takaori K, Nakamura J, Yamamoto S, Nakata H, Sato Y, Takase M, et al. Severity and frequency of proximal tubule injury determines renal prognosis. J Am Soc Nephrol. 2016;27:2393-2406. DOI: 10.1681/ASN.2015060647

[31] Duffield JS, Duffield JS. Cellular and molecular mechanisms in kidney fibrosis Find the latest version : Review series Cellular and molecular mechanisms in kidney fibrosis. J Clin Invest. 2014;124:2299-2306. DOI: 10.1172/JCI72267.a

[32] Yang L, Besschetnova TY, Brooks CR, Shah J V., Bonventre J V. Epithelial cell cycle arrest in G2/M mediates kidney fibrosis after injury. Nat Med. 2010;16:535-543. DOI: 10.1038/nm.2144

[33] He W, Dai C, Li Y, Zeng G, Monga SP, Liu Y. Wnt/ β-catenin signaling promotes renal interstitial fibrosis. J Am Soc Nephrol. 2009;20:765-776. DOI: 10.1681/ASN.2008060566

[34] Maarouf OH, Aravamudhan A, Rangarajan D, Kusaba T, Zhang V, Welborn J, et al. Paracrine wnt1 drives interstitial fibrosis without inflammation by tubulointerstitial cross-talk. J Am Soc Nephrol. 2016;27:781-790. DOI: 10.1681/ASN.2014121188

[35] Sato Y, Yanagita M. Renal anemia: from incurable to curable. Am J Physiol Renal Physiol. 2013;305:F1239-F1248. DOI: 10.1152/ajprenal.00233.2013

[36] Sugahara M, Tanaka T, Nangaku M. Prolyl hydroxylase domain inhibitors as a novel therapeutic approach against anemia in chronic kidney disease. Kidney Int. 2017;92:306-312. DOI: 10.1016/j.kint.2017.02.035

[37] Sato K, Kumagai N, Suzuki N. Alteration of the DNA Methylation Signature of Renal Erythropoietin-Producing Cells Governs the Sensitivity to Drugs Targeting the Hypoxia-Response Pathway in Kidney Disease Progression. Front Genet. 2019;10:1-8. DOI: 10.3389/fgene.2019.01134

[38] Chang YT, Yang CC, Pan SY, Chou YH, Chang FC, Lai CF, et al. DNA methyltransferase inhibition restores erythropoietin production in fibrotic murine kidneys. J Clin Invest. 2016;126:721-731. DOI: 10.1172/JCI82819

[39] Souma T, Nezu M, Nakano D, Yamazaki S, Hirano I, Sekine H, et al. Erythropoietin synthesis in renal myofibroblasts is restored by activation of hypoxia signaling. J Am Soc Nephrol. 2016;27:428-438. DOI: 10.1681/ASN.2014121184

[40] Fuchs MAA, Broeker KAE, Schrankl J, Burzlaff N, Willam C, Wagner C, et al. Inhibition of transforming growth factor β1 signaling in resident interstitial cells attenuates profibrotic gene expression and preserves erythropoietin production during experimental kidney fibrosis in mice. Kidney Int. 2021;1:10-14. DOI: 10.1016/j.kint.2021.02.035

[41] Zhu X, Perazella MA. HEMATOLOGY: ISSUES IN THE DIALYSIS PATIENT: Nonhematologic Complications of Erythropoietin Therapy. Semin Dial. 2006;19:279-284. DOI: 10.1111/j.1525-139x.2006.00173.x

[42] Chen N, Hao C, Peng X, Lin H, Yin A, Hao L, et al. Roxadustat for

Anemia in Patients with Kidney Disease Not Receiving Dialysis. N Engl J Med. 2019;381:1001-1010. DOI: 10.1056/nejmoa1813599

[43] Eckardt K-U, Agarwal R, Aswad A, Awad A, Block GA, Bacci MR, et al. Safety and Efficacy of Vadadustat for Anemia in Patients Undergoing Dialysis. N Engl J Med. 2021;384:1601-1612. DOI: 10.1056/nejmoa2025956

[44] Nangaku M, Hamano T, Akizawa T, Tsubakihara Y, Nagai R, Okuda N, et al. Daprodustat Compared with Epoetin Beta Pegol for Anemia in Japanese Patients Not on Dialysis: A 52-Week Randomized Open-Label Phase 3 Trial. Am J Nephrol. 2021;52:26-35. DOI: 10.1159/000513103

[45] Macdougall IC, Akizawa T, Berns JS, Bernhardt T, Krueger T. Effects of molidustat in the treatment of anemia in CKD. Clin J Am Soc Nephrol. 2019;14(1):28-39. DOI: 10.2215/CJN.02510218

[46] Nangaku M. Chronic hypoxia and tubulointerstitial injury: A final common pathway to end-stage renal failure. J Am Soc Nephrol. 2006;17:17-25. DOI: 10.1681/ASN.2005070757

[47] Schrimpf C, Teebken OE, Wilhelmi M, Duffield JS. The role of pericyte detachment in vascular rarefaction. J Vasc Res. 2014;51:247-258. DOI: 10.1159/000365149

[48] Norman JT, Orphanides C, Garcia P, Fine LG. Hypoxia-induced changes in extracellular matrix metabolism in renal cells. Exp Nephrol. 1999;7:463-469. DOI: 10.1159/000020625

[49] Zhang Y, Nakano D, Guan Y, Hitomi H, Uemura A, Masaki T, et al. A sodium-glucose cotransporter 2 inhibitor attenuates renal capillary injury and fibrosis by a vascular endothelial growth factor–dependent pathway after renal injury in mice. Kidney Int. 2018;94:524-535. DOI: 10.1016/j.kint.2018.05.002

[50] Sano M, Goto S. Possible mechanism of hematocrit elevation by sodium glucose cotransporter 2 inhibitors and associated beneficial renal and cardiovascular effects. Circulation. 2019;139:1985-1987. DOI: 10.1161/CIRCULATIONAHA.118.038881

[51] Lambers Heerspink HJ, Zeeuw D De, Wie L, Leslie B, List J. original article. Diabetes Obes Metab. 2013;159:853-862. DOI: 10.1111/dom.12127

[52] Nakamura J, Sato Y, Kitai Y, Wajima S, Yamamoto S, Oguchi A, et al. Myofibroblasts acquire retinoic acid–producing ability during fibroblast-to-myofibroblast transition following kidney injury. Kidney Int. 2019;95:526-539. DOI: 10.1016/j.kint.2018.10.017

[53] Schiessl IM, Grill A, Fremter K, Steppan D, Hellmuth MK, Castrop H. Renal interstitial platelet-derived growth factor receptor-β cells support proximal tubular regeneration. J Am Soc Nephrol. 2018;29:1383-1396. DOI: 10.1681/ASN.2017101069

[54] Leaf IA, Nakagawa S, Johnson BG, Cha JJ, Mittelsteadt K, Guckian KM, et al. Pericyte MyD88 and IRAK4 control inflammatory and fibrotic responses to tissue injury. J Clin Invest. 2017;127:321-334. DOI: 10.1172/JCI87532

[55] Perry HM, Görldt N, Sung SSJ, Huang L, Rudnicka KP, Encarnacion IM, et al. Perivascular CD73+ cells attenuate inflammation and interstitial fibrosis in the kidney microenvironment. Am J Physiol Renal Physiol. 2019;317:F658–F669. DOI: 10.1152/ajprenal.00243.2019

[56] Ishani A, Xue JL, Himmelfarb J, Eggers PW, Kimmel PL, Molitoris BA,

et al. Acute Kidney Injury Increases Risk of ESRD among Elderly. J Am Soc Nephrol. 2009;20:223-228. DOI: 10.1681/ASN.2007080837

[57] Luo S, Zhu R, Yu T, Fan H, Hu Y, Mohanta SK, et al. Chronic Inflammation: A Common Promoter in Tertiary Lymphoid Organ Neogenesis. Front Immunol. 2019;10:1-13. DOI: 10.3389/fimmu.2019.02938

[58] Pipi E, Nayar S, Gardner DH, Colafrancesco S, Smith C, Barone F. Tertiary lymphoid structures: Autoimmunity goes local. Front Immunol. 2018;9:1-21. DOI: 10.3389/fimmu.2018.01952

[59] Neyt K, Perros F, GeurtsvanKessel CH, Hammad H, Lambrecht BN. Tertiary lymphoid organs in infection and autoimmunity. Trends Immunol. 2012;33:297-305. DOI: 10.1016/j.it.2012.04.006

[60] Moyron-Quiroz JE, Rangel-Moreno J, Kusser K, Hartson L, Sprague F, Goodrich S, et al. Role of inducible bronchus associated lymphoid tissue (iBALT) in respiratory immunity. Nat Med. 2004;10:927-934. DOI: 10.1038/nm1091

[61] Heesters BA, Myers RC, Carroll MC. Follicular dendritic cells: Dynamic antigen libraries. Nat Rev Immunol. 2014;14:495-504. DOI: 10.1038/nri3689

[62] Pei G, Zeng R, Han M, Liao P, Zhou X, Li Y, et al. Renal interstitial infiltration and tertiary lymphoid organ neogenesis in IgA nephropathy. Clin J Am Soc Nephrol. 2014;9:255-264. DOI: 10.2215/CJN.01150113

[63] Chang A, Henderson SG, Brandt D, Liu N, Guttikonda R, Hsieh C, et al. In Situ B Cell-Mediated Immune Responses and Tubulointerstitial Inflammation in Human Lupus Nephritis. J Immunol. 2011;186:1849-1860. DOI: 10.4049/jimmunol.1001983

[64] Miyanaga T, Mizuguchi K, Hara S, Zoshima T, Inoue D, Nishioka R, et al. Tertiary lymphoid tissue in early-stage IgG4-related tubulointerstitial nephritis incidentally detected with a tumor lesion of the ureteropelvic junction: a case report. BMC Nephrol. 2021;22:1-7. DOI: 10.1186/s12882-021-02240-1

[65] Thaunat O, Patey N, Caligiuri G, Gautreau C, Mamani-Matsuda M, Mekki Y, et al. Chronic Rejection Triggers the Development of an Aggressive Intragraft Immune Response through Recapitulation of Lymphoid Organogenesis. J Immunol. 2010;185:717-728. DOI: 10.4049/jimmunol.0903589

[66] Sato Y, Boor P, Fukuma S, Klinkhammer BM, Haga H, Ogawa O, et al. Developmental stages of tertiary lymphoid tissue reflect local injury and inflammation in mouse and human kidneys. Kidney Int. 2020;98:448-463. DOI: 10.1016/j.kint.2020.02.023

Chapter 5

Fibroblast-Like Synovial Cell Subsets in Rheumatoid Arthritis

Søren Lomholt, Morten A. Nielsen, Maithri P. Aspari, Peter B. Jørgensen, Adam P. Croft, Christopher Buckley and Tue W. Kragstrup

Abstract

Fibroblasts like synoviocytes (FLS) play several significant roles in rheumatoid arthritis (RA) pathophysiology. This chapter will describe known roles of FLS in disease initiation, joint inflammation, disease persistence and joint destruction. It will describe the newly characterized subsets of FLS based on single cell RNA sequencing studies, and their association to specific aspects of the disease. Finally, we will discuss the future of targeting FLS in the treatment of RA. The FLS in the synovial lining layer are identified by surface complement decay-accelerating factor (CD55) along with lubricin and metallopeptidase expression. Pathological activation of this lining layer subset result in bone and cartilage damage in mice. FLS of the sublining layer are often characterized by THY1 expression, but recent studies have highlighted a heterogeneity where several distinct subsets are identified by additional markers. Sublining FLS expressing human leukocyte antigen-DRA (HLA-DRA) produce C-X-C motif chemokine 12 (CXCL12) and receptor activator of nuclear factor-κB ligand (RANKL) and seems to constitute a pro-inflammatory subset that is associated with inflammation and tertiary lymphoid structures. Another subset of FLS characterized by CD34 expression may discriminate a common progenitor fibroblast subset. Taken together, studies isolating and characterizing gene expression in synovial FLS report both associations of unknown importance and markers that may impose protective or destructive features. This supports evidence of FLS as active players in RA pathology capable of cellular recruitment, local cellular crosstalk and promotion of joint destruction. These discoveries may serve as an atlas for synovial activation in RA and have identified several potential fibroblast markers for the development of targeted treatment.

Keywords: Fibroblast like synoviocytes, Rheumatoid arthritis, Inflammation, Autoimmunity, Tertiary lymphoid structures, Fibroblast activation protein, Fibroblast targeted treatment

1. Introduction

In normal resting conditions the synovial membrane is a thin layer of well-ordered cells historically called type A and B synoviocytes. These cells form a barrier between the articular cavity and a sublining layer, the latter being heterogeneous and composed of several cell linages. Fibroblasts, immune cells and mature vasculature (capillaries, arterioles and venules) made up of pericytes and endothelia are some of the various cell types constituting this layer [1–3].

2. Rheumatoid arthritis

Rheumatoid arthritis (RA) has a multifactorial etiology and is one among the most common systemic autoimmune diseases [4, 5]. The factors that mediate the initiation of RA is yet to be unraveled. However, the pathology of RA involves abnormalities in both the innate and the adaptive immune system, and both of these systems are implicated with the progression and persistence of the disease [6, 7]. The synovial membrane is the primary site of pathology during the synovitis stage of the disease and characterized by proliferation of tissue resident, synovial cells and the infiltration of inflammatory cells from the blood. RA is a chronic, progressive disease leading to degradation of articular cartilage and bone along with several systemic manifestations [8].

In RA, the inflamed synovial membrane undergoes hyperplasia and transforms into less structured lining layer and sublining tissues both rich in fibroblasts like synoviocytes (FLS) [9, 10]. This inflamed synovial membrane eventually begins to invade the cartilage surfaces and the underlying bone, commonly referred to as pannus [11, 12].

Present day treatment strategies for RA primarily focuses on suppression of cytokine signaling and T- and B-cell activity. These therapies have highlighted the importance of immune response in driving the progression of RA. However, they also clearly demonstrate that in a large proportion of patients these treatments are incapable of inducing disease remission [8, 13]. Synovial phenotyping of RA patients based on histology has highlighted a fibroblast dominated synovial pathotype [14]. This pathotype is believed to include a large proportion of the non-responders to conventional and biologic disease modifying anti-rheumatic drugs [15–17]. This is supported *in vitro* where anti-tumor necrosis factor alpha (TNFα) treatments were ineffective in cultures dominated by FLS [18]. Furthermore, a recently published, biopsy driven clinical trial in RA patients with inadequate response to anti-TNFα treatment, showed significantly higher response rates when patients with B-cell poor synovium were treated with IL-6 receptor inhibitor tocilizumab compared to the B-cell depleting agent rituximab [19].

In the following sections, we will first describe RA FLS in general before the era of single cell RNA sequencing (scRNA-seq). We will summarize the known and proposed roles of FLS in RA initiation, joint inflammation, disease persistence and joint destruction. Finally, we will describe the newly characterized subsets of FLS based on scRNA-seq studies their connection to specific aspects of clinical disease, future outlooks in the context of RA diagnosis, RA tissue phenotyping and therapy targeting FLS.

3. Fibroblast like synovial cells in rheumatoid arthritis

3.1 Disease initiation

The central role of FLS in RA pathology is highlighted in murine studies demonstrating that activation of FLS is sufficient to initiate local joint inflammation leading to persistent arthritis [20, 21].

Furthermore, FLS greatly contribute to the transformation of the thin synovial membrane into a multi-layered invasive hyperplastic pannus [22]. This expansion of FLS in the inflamed synovium is likely a result of at least one of the following processes. First, pathological subsets of FLS seem to proliferate to some extent and develop a local resistance to apoptosis [23–25]. Secondly, pluripotent mesenchymal stem cells may migrate into the synovium from the circulation, where they differentiate into mature pathological subsets of FLS [26]. Lastly, a local mesenchymal progenitor cell population may undergo activation and differentiation into distinct phenotypes of FLS [27]. Collectively, this leads to a local increase in pathological FLS in the RA synovium.

3.2 Joint inflammation

Pathogenic FLS constitute the majority of cells found in the inflamed synovial tissues, and play an important role in the inflammatory cascade, linking innate and adaptive immunity [6, 10]. FLS are capable of significantly affecting the local inflamed environment through production of cytokines and chemokines leading to recruitment and activation of immune cells [9, 28]. Specifically, pathogenic FLS are able to provide an adequate survival signal for synovial T-cells [29], a signal that is superior to the one produced by non-inflammatory fibroblasts [30]. This interaction between FLS and lymphocytes can inhibit the resolution of local inflammation [30, 31] through both paracrine and direct cell–cell interactions [32]. This pathogenic role of the FLS is facilitated by the up-regulation of several adhesion molecules such as intercellular adhesion molecule 1 (ICAM-1) and vascular cell adhesion molecule 1 (VCAM-1) [6, 33]. In addition to recruitment and co-activation of T-cells in the inflamed joint, FLS have been shown to be able to present antigens on class II major histocompatibility complex (MHC-II) to CD4+ T-cells [34].

Furthermore, FLS are involved in the formation of tertiary lymphoid structures (TLS) in the RA synovium. Stromal cell populations such as the fibroblastic reticular cell support organization of these lymphocyte aggregates similarly to that of secondary lymphoid organs with distinct T- and B-cell niches [35]. Thymocyte differentiation antigen 1 (THY1, also known as CD90) and podoplanin (PDPN) positive fibroblast associated with TLS in RA (**Table 1**) produce several chemokines such as C-X-C motif ligand (CXCL) 13 and C-C motif ligand (CCL)21 implicated with lymphocyte recruitment and organization [47, 48]. Another marker associated with the TLS associated fibroblast is the receptor activator of nuclear factor kappa-β ligand (RANKL), which is important in both bone homeostasis and lymph node development [35, 49].

Collectively, FLS may be involved in both the pro-inflammatory initiation in the synovium, lymphocyte recruitment and the organization of TLS. A fibroblast driven RA phenotype resulting in persistent inflammation and a lymphoid rich synovium similar to what have been shown by histology.

3.3 Disease persistence

The highly proliferating and pathogenic RA FLS are very different from their quiescent state during non-inflamed conditions where FLS control the structural integrity of the joint lining and sublining layer [22]. The immunological events initiating a pathogenic state of RA FLS is still not fully understood, but proliferation and transformation of the FLS may occur prior to immune infiltration [50].

In RA, subsets of FLS can differentiate to become inflammatory, migratory, and invasive, thus collectively fostering disease aggravation in various animal models of RA [45, 51, 52]. Constitutive activation is a hallmark of RA FLS and leads to production of several inflammatory cytokines, such as interleukin (IL)-1β, TNFα and IL-6 and chemokines such as monocyte chemoattractant protein 1 (MCP-1/CLL2) [9] and CXCL12 [53]. Even though the activation of RA FLS is greatly affected by pro-inflammatory factors in the local environment, epigenetic changes are also important [54]. Epigenetic changes lead to constitutive activation even when the cells are removed from the inflamed environment and remain without addition of proinflammatory stimuli [52]. Moreover, a

Classical synovial subsets in RA	**Markers**		
Fibroblast like synoviocytes [36–38]	Vimentin, THY1, prolyl-5-hydroxylase, CDH11, CD45, HLA-DR, α-SMA, CD55		
Macrophage like synoviocytes [36, 39–41]	CD14, CD68, RFD7, CD163, CD206, HLA-DR, CD97		
Tertiary lymphoid structure associated fibroblast [35]	PDPN, THY1, FAP, CXCL13, CCL21, RANKL, CD21		
Fibrocyte [42]	CD34, CD45, CD14, CD11, MHC-II		
Single cell analysis of synovial fibroblast subsets in RA			
Published studies and subsets	**Cluster markers**	**Associated transcription profile**	
Stephenson et al. 2018 [43]	Fibroblast sorting strategy: CD45 - Propidium iodide - PDPN+		
Sublining fibroblast	THY1+		
Lining fibroblast	CD55+	HAS1	
Mizoguchi et al. 2018 [44]	Fibroblast sorting strategy: CD45- CD31- CD235a- CD146- PDPN+		
Perivascular fibroblast	THY1+ CD34-	RANKL^{high}, OPG^{low}	Migration factors: CTHRC1, TWIST1, POSTN, LOXL2, PDGFBB, MMP14
Sublining fibroblast	CD34+	IL6, CXCL12, CCL2, OPG	
Lining fibroblast	THY1- CD34-	CD55, PRG4, HAS1, MMP1, MMP3	
Zhang et al. 2019 [10]	Fibroblast sorting strategy: CD45- CD31- PDPN+		
SC-F1 (sublining)	THY1+ CD34+	C3, FOS	
SC-F2 (sublining)	THY1+ HLA-DRA^{high}	IL6, CXCL12	
SC-F3 (sublining)	THY1+ DKK3+	CADM1, COL8A2	
SC-F4 (lining)	THY1- CD55+	PRG4, HBEGF, CLIC5	
Croft et al. 2019 [45]	Reanalysis of human data from Zhang et al. [10].		
F1 (sublining)	THY1+	DKK3, OGN, CD9,	
F2 (sublining)	THY1+	MDK, COL8A1, AEBP1	
F3 (sublining)	THY1+	IRF1, EGR1, JUNB	
F4 (lining)	THY1-	CLIC5, CD55, HBEGF	
F5 (sublining)	CD34+	C3, APOD	
Single cell analysis of circulating mesenchymal cells in RA:			
Published study and subset	**Associated transcription profile**		
Orange et al. 2020 [46]	Fibroblast sorting strategy: CD45- CD31- PDPN+		
AC3 (sublining fibroblast phenotype)	CD34, HLA-DR, DKK3, FAPα, CDH11		

The table contains a list of surface and transcriptional profiles of fibroblast subsets, fibroblast like cell subsets and macrophage subsets (pre-scRNA-seq) related to rheumatoid arthritis. For scRNA-seq studies, fibroblast subset names refer to the original articles. "+" and "- "shows whether the cells of interest are positive or negative for the cellular markers. The cellular markers which are discussed in the text are also listed under abbreviations.

Table 1.
Surface and transcriptional profiles of FLS subsets (and related cellular subsets) in rheumatoid arthritis.

recent study suggests a link between epigenetic-driven positional identity of FLS (e.g. small versus large joints and proximal versus distal joints) and clinical disease patterns [55]. This link is further supported by the finding of oncogenes at sites of tissue destruction [56, 57] together with a highly activated nuclear factor κ beta pathway in RA FLS [58].

Altered metabolic activity with increased glycolysis is another hallmark of RA FLS [59]. Metabolic reprogramming of FLS were recently connected to complement

C3 and C3a receptor-activation. Here repeated inflammatory challenges resulted in a distinct pro-inflammatory phenotypic priming of FLS in mice models of arthritis [60].

On the opposite side, several factors attempt to facilitate remission of proinflammatory FLS. One such potential immune regulator is the MerTK expressing synovial macrophage which *in vitro* reduce matrix metalloproteinase (MMP) production by lining layer FLS [61].

Thus, even though FLS are responsive to their inflammatory context they may possess a distinct positional identity which enables a cytokine-independent intrinsic activation contributing to disease persistence in RA.

3.4 Joint destruction

The severe joint destruction of late-stage RA is in part attributed to the pannus tissue which is rich in FLS. RA FLS are identified as invaders of the joint cartilage *in vivo* [62, 63], an invasive behavior that has been confirmed *in vitro* [64] and in mice [52]. FLS mediate cartilage degradation which is attributed to a combination of facilitating adhesion factors and production of proteases, here among several well-known matrix metalloproteinases (MMPs) [9, 52, 64]. Cartilage degradation is ameliorated when fibroblast activation protein (FAP) deficiency is induced in the human TNFα transgenic mice model of arthritis [65]. The invasiveness of pathological RA FLS is further emphasized by human FLS migrating to other joints in mouse models of RA and degrading the implanted human cartilage [51]. Migration that may be facilitated by specific anticitrulinated protein antibodies [66]. Notably, the *ex vivo* invasiveness of FLS correlates with joint erosions [67].

Increased osteoclastic activity leading to bone erosions in RA is another major factor in joint destruction. Here FLS produce CXCL12, RANKL, dickkopf related protein (DKK) 1, etc. which may increase both osteoclast migration, differentiation, proliferation/activation and inhibit osteoblast function [53, 68, 69].

4. Single cell analysis of synovial fibroblast subsets in rheumatoid arthritis

4.1 Phenotyping of fibroblast like synovial cells

Increasing spatial and molecular resolution in present day cellular analysis are changing our view of the synovial membrane in RA. Most notable is the identification of different fibroblast subsets within the inflamed synovial membrane. Recent work and ongoing studies are utilizing scRNA-seq, CyTOF and flow cytometry cell sorting to further investigate and distinguish these subsets and their role in disease pathology.

Recent scRNA-seq studies have identified several distinct disease-associated subsets in the inflamed synovial membrane, often grouped as lining layer or sublining layer FLS [10, 43, 44], **Figure 1**. The present studies utilize flow cytometry assisted cell sorting and transcriptomic clustering strategies based on exclusion of hematopoietic lineage cells (CD45), endothelial cells (CD31), red blood cells (CD235a), and pericytes (CD146) while using PDPN or collagen production as a positive marker (**Table 1**).

4.2 Lining layer fibroblasts

A common finding in scRNA-seq studies confirms the presence of complement decay-accelerating factor (CD55) and absence of THY1 expression in FLS of the

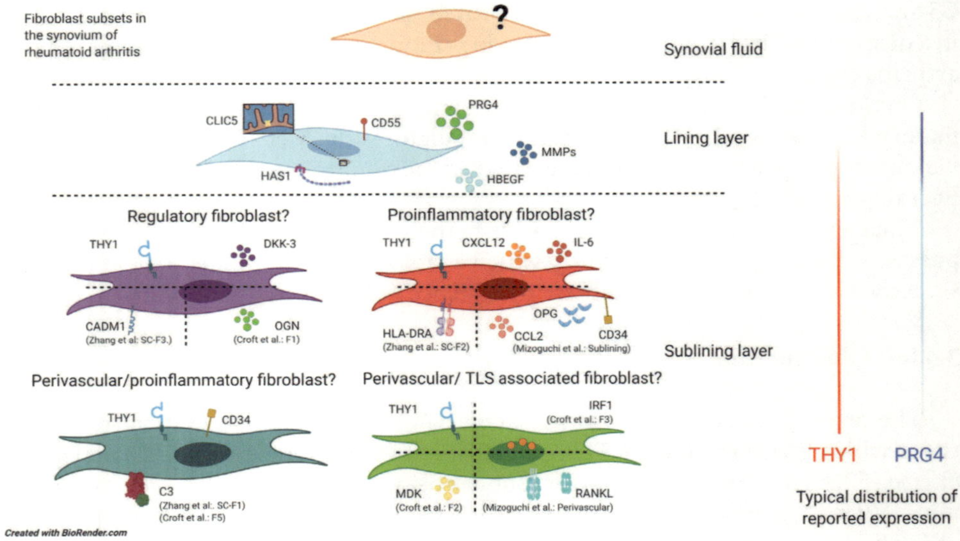

Figure 1.
The figure is a schematic presentation of fibroblast subsets identified by scRNA-seq studies of synovial tissue from patients with rheumatoid arthritis. The subsets have been divided into lining layer FLS and sublining layer FLS. No scRNA-seq studies yet have examined fibroblast subsets from the synovial fluid. Based on grouping markers and transcription profiles listed in ***Table 1****, we propose 4 sublining phenotypes. Cells have been divided by dashed lines when the cellular markers were not listed in all the original studies. THY-1 and PRG4 expression gradients from the lining layer to the sublining layer is shown by the color density of the red and blue bars. The cellular markers are discussed in the text and listed under abbreviations. TLS: Tertiary lymphoid structures.*

lining layer (**Table 1**). Of note, Mizoguchi et al. [44] did not report histological data of CD55 distribution, but a high level of CD55 gene expression in CD34- THY1- lining layer fibroblasts. All scRNA-seq studies (**Table 1**) of joint tissue reported lubricin (PRG4) expression in the lining layer subset [10, 43–45]. All present studies showed similar patterns of gene expression pertaining to the potential markers of FLS presented in the following section.

Zhang et al. [10] and the reanalysis of the same human data by Croft et al. [45] both reported a distinct lining fibroblast subset, SC-F4 and F4 respectively. This lining fibroblast subset was associated with expression of chloride intracellular ion channel 5 (CLIC5) and heparin binding epidermal growth factor-like growth factor (HBEGF). Mizoguchi et al. [44] and Stephenson et al. [43] also reported increased hyaluronan synthase 1 (HAS1) and metallopeptidase expression.

HAS1 is important for hyaluronan production and is a response to pro-inflammatory stimuli in RA synoviocytes. This activation results in hyaluronan cell coating, leukocyte/monocyte recruitment and facilitation of fibroblast-monocytes binding [70].

CD55, a C3 convertase inhibitor, has received increasing interest in cancer, where CD55/CD97 binding is associated with several oncogenic properties such as invasion and migration [71]. In RA, CD55 positive FLS are exclusive to the lining layer and in proximity to CD97 positive macrophages, suggesting a possible mechanism of crosstalk [36]. CD55 is not exclusive to RA [72], but it has been suggested as a protective factor in a mice model of immune complex mediated arthritis [73].

In the context of joint tissue, the mucin-like glycoprotein, PRG4, has been proposed as having a dual role comprising of well-known lubricating property and as a moderator of inflammation via NF-κβ pathways through interaction with both CD44 and toll-like receptors [74].

CLIC5 is present in several intracellular organelles, but predominantly located at the mitochondrial inner membrane, where it has been associated with modulation of reactive oxygen species [75]. However, no functional studies have been published regarding CLIC5 in RA.

The epidermal growth factor family member, HBEGF, is present and involved in several physiological processes such as wound healing, tumor formation and angiogenesis. One common topic is its association with cell migration, as seen in keratinocyte/fibroblast models and in enterocytes in necrotizing enterocolitis [76]. In RA, HBEGF positive macrophages have recently been shown to increase synovial fibroblast invasiveness in an *in vitro* model [77].

Several matrix metalloproteinases, MMP1, MMP3 and MMP14 was connected to a specific subset of FLS by Mizoguchi et al. [44]. These destructive enzymes have previously been connected to cartilage degradation in RA, but MMP14 was also noted by Mizoguchi et al. as a migratory factor [44].

Taken together, studies isolating and characterizing gene expression in lining layer fibroblasts report both associations of unknown importance and markers that may impose protective and destructive features. This suggests that the lining layer fibroblast subset is an active subset in RA pathology capable of cellular recruitment and significant local cellular crosstalk.

4.3 Sublining layer fibroblasts

The scRNA-seq studies have reported several distinct sublining subsets presented in **Table 1**. The initial study by Stephenson et al. [43] identified THY1 as a marker of sublining fibroblasts and the subsequent scRNA-seq studies confirmed THY1 as a specific, albeit not universal marker of sublining fibroblasts [10, 44, 45].

Zhang et al. characterized this heterogeneity of the sublining layer fibroblasts and defined three THY1+ groups with additional subset markers; CD34 defined the SC-F1 cluster, human leukocyte antigen (HLA)-DRA^{high} defined the SC-F2 cluster and DKK-3 defined the SC-F3 cluster. The SC-F2 in particular was significantly increased in leukocyte-rich RA ssynovium compared to leukocyte-poor RA synovium and osteoarthritis (OA) synovium [10], suggesting these to encompass TLS-associated fibroblast subsets. Reanalysis of these human data by Croft et al. [45] enabled the distinction of four sublining layer fibroblast groups (F1–3,-5, **Table 1**).

As with the lining layer, large sets of multiomics data are available. Several markers connected to joint inflammation and destruction have been identified in these subsets. However, the markers most consistently reported are THY1, HLA-DRA, CD34, DKK3.

THY1 is a glycoprotein present on the membrane of several different cells including endothelial and mesenchymal cells [78]. Among the functions associated with THY1 expression is cellular contact, CD97 binding, integrin binding, trans-endothelial migration and MMP-9 and CXCL8 secretion after binding to neutrophiles [78].

As with THY1, CD34 is an established marker in different cell types including several stromal cells, epi/endothelial cells and fibrocytes [79]. Its function is largely unknown but has been linked to proliferation, adhesion, differentiation and is proposed as a marker of progenitor subsets in both mesenchymal, epithelial and endothelial cells [79].

MHC molecule (both class I and II) functions are typically attributed to antigen presentation. Several MHC molecules have been associated with autoimmune disease. Examples are the association of the MHC-I molecule HLA-B27 with ankylosing spondylitis, reactive arthritis and juvenile idiopathic arthritis subsets [80], and the association of MHC-II molecules HLA-DR1 and DR4 association with RA [81]. The specific function of HLA-DRA in RA FLS is yet to be investigated.

The DKK family of glycoproteins are well known modulators of WNT pathways connected to embryogenesis, bone formation and eye and skin development [82]. DKK-1 has been extensively described in fibroblasts from RA patients and is a key player in joint remodeling [69]. DKK-3 has been reported as a chondroprotective factor in OA [83] and suggested as a B-cell modulator whose absence aggravates autoimmune symptoms in a murine systemic lupus erythematosus model [84] and a CD8 T-cell modulator involved in antigen tolerance [85].

Enrichment of several genes related to pro-inflammatory cytokines and proteins related to bone metabolism in RA have been reported in sublining fibroblasts including IL-6, MCP-1/CCL2, CXCL12 and RANKL. Two proteins not mentioned above is the RANKL decoy receptor osteoprotegerin (OPG) which inhibit osteoclastogenesis in synovial macrophages [86] and the relatively new osteoglycin (OGN) that may both be part of the vascular system and may affect osteoblast differentiation [87].

The interferon regulatory factor 1 (IRF1) is a significant component of the interferon signature/inflammation pathway, through which TNF induces production of CXCL9–11 and in its absence diminishes B-cell activating factor expression [88].

The heparin-binding growth factor midkine (MDK) is less investigated than the above-mentioned cytokines but has been identified in human synoviocytes and associated with leukocyte migration to the synovium and osteoclastogenesis in mice [89].

C3, a unifying step for all three complement activating pathways has previously been located around microvasculature in the sublining of the RA synovium [90].

The cellular adhesion molecule 1 (CADM1) is a transmembrane member of the immunoglobulin superfamily with no known relation to RA. It has been identified as a tumor suppressor gene in solid cancers such as squamous cell carcinoma a, but may contribute to infiltration in adult T-cell leukemia/lymphoma [91].

To summarize, the sublining layer is a heterogeneous compartment of the inflamed RA synovium, regarding both cell linages and especially fibroblast subsets (**Table 1** and **Figure 1**). Several distinct fibroblast subsets have been identified, but recuring markers such as HLA-DRA, CD34 and DKK-3 are relatively unknown in the RA context. Results from scRNA-seq studies propose that the sublining layer fibroblast subsets are significantly involved in cellular crosstalk, leukocyte recruitment, para- and autocrine pro-inflammatory stimulation, and joint tissue destruction. Notably, some distinguishing factors such as DKK-3 may be enriched to form a regulatory anti-inflammatory and pro self-tolerance subset with similar chondroprotective effects and immune modulation of antigen tolerance mentioned in the previous section. An HLA-DRA^{high}/CXCL12/RANKL^{high} associated subset may constitute the pro-inflammatory TLS associated fibroblast subsets and CD34 may discriminate a common progenitor fibroblast subset. Together, the presence of both pro-inflammatory subsets and potential anti-inflammatory and progenitor subsets suggests an ongoing cellular balancing throughout the sublining layer, which may open avenues for new research in treatment strategies targeting FLS.

4.4 Fibroblast like synoviocytes in rheumatoid arthritis compared to other arthritides

In RA, synovial division into lining/sublining layers suggests differentiated roles of subsets of FLS regarding cytokine production, joint destruction, and possible regulatory mechanisms.

The expansion of these distinct subsets is different in RA compared with OA. Mizoguchi et al. reported a greater fraction of the THY1^{+} CD34^{-} (perivascular) subset but less of the THY1^{-} CD34^{-} (lining) subset in RA compared with OA [44]. Notably, here the proportion of THY1^{+} CD34^{-} (perivascular) FLS correlated with leukocyte infiltration and ultrasonic and histological synovitis [44].

Similarly, Zhang et al. reported an overabundance of the THY1$^+$ CD34$^-$ HLA-DRA^{high} (SC-F2) subset with upregulated expression of CXCL12 and IL-6 and a THY1$^+$ CD34$^+$ (SC-F1) subset in RA. In contrast, lining FLS (SC-F4) were more fabundant in OA [10].

The causal link between distinct subsets and RA pathogenesis was investigated in mice by Croft et al. Here the mouse thy1$^-$ subset homologous to human lining FLS (F4) were correlated to joint damage and mouse thy1$^+$ sublining FLS correlated to inflammation [45]. Notably, the elimination of FAP expressing subsets reduced pannus formation and joint destruction [45]. This suggests that FAP is a marker of pathologically active FLS in RA [45, 92, 93].

Comparison of subsets of FLS in RA and psoriatic arthritis are underway [94] and may potentially assist in discriminating these arthritides.

5. Fibroblasts derived from synovial fluid versus synovial tissue

Arthrocentesis is a common therapeutic procedure in treatment of RA. Fibroblast cultured from synovial fluid aspirates initially express similar phenotypical traits compared to tissue derived synovial fibroblast cultures [95, 96]. Despite these similarities, synovial fluid derived fibroblasts are likely a proxy regarding changes in the synovium and results must be interpreted as such. In both research and clinical settings synovial biopsies are both economical and well tolerated [97–100]. However, synovial fluid analysis of both cellular and soluble components is very useful in clinical settings where the length of consultations/sterile procedural environments/analytic facilities may limit the use of synovial biopsies. To the authors knowledge, no studies have yet reported scRNA-seq analysis of synovial fluid fibroblasts.

6. Circulating mesenchymal fibroblast like cells in rheumatoid arthritis

In excess to tissue resident FLS, Orange et al. recently highlighted the presence of circulating fibroblast-like cells in the blood of RA patients shortly before symptomatic disease flare [46]. Interestingly these pre inflammatory mesenchymal (PRIME) cells show enrichment of previously reported markers of distinct sublining subsets of FLS e.g., DKK-3, CD34 and HLA-DR. This suggests that PRIME cells may constitute a heterogeneous pool of circulating FLS-like cells with distinct functions. Subsets of FLS migrating from the RA affected synovium, or a common homogeneous pool of circulating progenitor FLS awaiting recruitment signals from local sites of inflammation could potentially be the origin of these cells, although this remains to be investigated. Regardless, PRIME cells may not only be a useful marker predicting disease flares in RA, but also potentially explain how synovitis is transmitted from joint to joint [51].

7. Future therapeutic perspectives

The insights recently generated through high resolution scRNA-seq have revolutionized our understanding of specific subsets of FLS in RA and their involvement in driving different aspects of RA pathobiology. This understanding has also provided the basis for generating specific targetable markers of pathological subsets of FLS in RA. Targeting strategies that could be used as either monotherapy or as an add-on treatment to present day cytokine or lymphocyte inhibitors [101].

FLS could be targeted by drugs used in fibrotic conditions such as nintedanib or pirfenidone [102]. However, these drugs are likely affecting a completely different aspect of fibroblast functions. Therefore, new drugs are needed. An example is the addition of the cyclin-dependent kinase inhibitor, Seliciclib, which is currently being evaluated [103].

The well-known FAP marker of activated stromal cells has a diagnostic and prognostic potential through precise and low background positron emission tomography tracers developed in cancer-immunology [104]. The recent development of specific quinoline-based positron emission tomography tracers that act as FAP inhibitors have demonstrated promising results both preclinically and clinically in different cancers but could also be promising as diagnostic and prognostic markers of RA [105]. Further, the clinical potential of targeting FAP expressing FLS would be a targeted treatment eliminating pathologically activated RA FLS, in both the lining and the sublining layer [45, 93].

Among other interesting targets, NOTCH3 is one of the most recently *in vivo* validated pathological targets. NOTCH3 is expressed on the surface of RA FLS and linked with THY1 expression. NOTCH3 may also be a useful target in a therapeutic senescence strategy through selective activation of the g-protein coupled receptor melanocontin type 1 receptor [106]. Furthermore, in an animal model of RA injection of NOTCH3-neutralizing monoclonal antibody attenuated the severity of arthritis. Taken together, the *in vitro* studies on NOTCH3, including its connection to spatial distribution of FLS and the above-mentioned animal study underline NOTCH3 as a promising therapeutical target in RA [106, 107]. Targeting the complement C3 - C3a receptor axis may serve as another preventive or complementary strategy, where metabolic priming of FLS can be avoided or reduced [60]. Another possible strategy of targeting FLS is drug delivery via the extra domain A fibronectin splice variant identified in OA and RA [108, 109] and utilized in cancer [110].

Several other reagents targeting FLS are currently being tested ranging from metabolite modulators to treatments targeting intracellular signal transduction or epigenetic changes [111].

Collectively, these therapies targeting subsets of FLS are emerging as promising diagnostic and therapeutic tools. Tools for optimized and stratified treatments in RA based on which cellular mechanisms and which fibroblast subsets are pathologically activated in the individual patient.

8. Conclusions

Collectively, pathological FLS presented in this chapter are deeply connected to the RA pathophysiology of disease initiation, joint inflammation, disease persistence and joint tissue destruction.

Recent scRNA-seq studies have identified several distinct subsets of FLS causally linked to major elements of RA pathogenesis e.g., inflammation and joint destruction, while other subsets may present regulatory, pro-inflammatory TLS associated or common progenitor FLS.

These first steps in a scRNA-seq era of RA research warrants both rejoice and due diligence. Due diligence because we henceforth must appreciate the cellular diversity and the complex cellular crosstalk of the RA synovium. Like FLS, monocytes/macrophages and lymphocytes exhibit distinct subsets in RA, which may be as important in understanding the spectrum of RA disease, e.g., lymphocyte dominated vs. lymphocyte poor synovium and erosive vs. non-erosive disease. Furthermore, we must appreciate the heterogeneity of FLS and cellular organization (here among TLS formation) of the sublining layer.

Rejoice because the recent subset studies have produced a language and knowledge and a novel nomenclature for FLS in future research. A breakthrough that might enable clinicians in the future to modulate specific aspects of RA through fibroblast subset targeted treatment.

Conflict of interest

The authors declare no conflict of interest.

Abbreviations

RA	Rheumatoid arthritis
FLS	Fibroblast like synoviocytes
TNFα	Tumor necrosis factor alpha
scRNA-seq	Single cell RNA sequencing
ICAM-1	Intercellular adhesion molecule 1
VCAM-1	Vascular cell adhesion molecule 1
MHC-II	Type 2 major histocompadability complex
TLS	Tertiary lymphoid structures
THY1	Thymocyte differentiation antigen 1
PDPN	Podoplanin
CXCL	C-X-C motif ligand
CCL	C-C motif ligand
RANKL	Receptor activator of nuclear factor kappa-β ligand
IL	Interleukin
MCP-1/CLL2	Monocyte chemoattractant protein 1
MMP	Matrix metalloproteinases
FAP	Fibroblast activation protein
DKK	Dickkopf related protein
CD55	Complement decay-accelerating factor
PRG4	Lubricin
CLIC5	Chloride intracellular ion channel 5
HBEGF	Heparin binding epidermal growth factor-like growth factor
HLA	Human leukocyte antigen
OA	Osteoarthritis
OPG	Osteoprotegerin
OGN	Osteoglycin
IRF1	Interferon regulatory factor 1
MDK	Midkine
CADM1	Cellular adhesion molecule 1

Author details

Søren Lomholt[1], Morten A. Nielsen[1], Maithri P. Aspari[1], Peter B. Jørgensen[2], Adam P. Croft[3], Christopher Buckley[3] and Tue W. Kragstrup[1*]

1 Department of Biomedicine, Aarhus University, Aarhus, Denmark

2 Section for Immunology, Technical University of Denmark, Denmark

3 Rheumatology Research Group, University of Birmingham, Birmingham, UK

*Address all correspondence to: kragstrup@biomed.au.dk

References

[1] Castor CW. The microscopic structure of normal human synovial tissue. Arthritis and rheumatism. 1960;3:140-51.

[2] Kennedy A, Ng CT, Biniecka M, Saber T, Taylor C, O'Sullivan J, et al. Angiogenesis and blood vessel stability in inflammatory arthritis. Arthritis and rheumatism. 2010;62(3):711-21.

[3] Culemann S, Grüneboom A, Nicolás-Ávila J, Weidner D, Lämmle KF, Rothe T, et al. Locally renewing resident synovial macrophages provide a protective barrier for the joint. Nature. 2019;572(7771):670-5.

[4] Cooper GS, Stroehla BC. The epidemiology of autoimmune diseases. Autoimmun Rev. 2003;2(3):119-25.

[5] Gabriel SE, Michaud K. Epidemiological studies in incidence, prevalence, mortality, and comorbidity of the rheumatic diseases. Arthritis research & therapy. 2009;11(3):229.

[6] Cooles FA, Isaacs JD. Pathophysiology of rheumatoid arthritis. Current opinion in rheumatology. 2011;23(3):233-40.

[7] Burmester GR, Feist E, Dörner T. Emerging cell and cytokine targets in rheumatoid arthritis. Nature reviews Rheumatology. 2014;10(2):77-88.

[8] McInnes IB, Schett G. Pathogenetic insights from the treatment of rheumatoid arthritis. Lancet. 2017;389(10086):2328-37.

[9] Bartok B, Firestein GS. Fibroblast-like synoviocytes: key effector cells in rheumatoid arthritis. Immunol Rev. 2010;233(1):233-55.

[10] Zhang F, Wei K, Slowikowski K, Fonseka CY, Rao DA, Kelly S, et al. Defining inflammatory cell states in rheumatoid arthritis joint synovial tissues by integrating single-cell transcriptomics and mass cytometry. Nature immunology. 2019;20(7):928-42.

[11] Firestein GS. Evolving concepts of rheumatoid arthritis. Nature. 2003;423(6937):356-61.

[12] Shiozawa S, Shiozawa K, Fujita T. Morphologic observations in the early phase of the cartilage-pannus junction. Light and electron microscopic studies of active cellular pannus. Arthritis and rheumatism. 1983;26(4):472-8.

[13] Atzeni F, Sarzi-Puttini P, Gorla R, Marchesoni A, Caporali R. Switching rheumatoid arthritis treatments: an update. Autoimmun Rev. 2011;10(7):397-403.

[14] Dennis G, Jr., Holweg CT, Kummerfeld SK, Choy DF, Setiadi AF, Hackney JA, et al. Synovial phenotypes in rheumatoid arthritis correlate with response to biologic therapeutics. Arthritis research & therapy. 2014;16(2):R90.

[15] Pitzalis C, Kelly S, Humby F. New learnings on the pathophysiology of RA from synovial biopsies. Current opinion in rheumatology. 2013;25(3):334-44.

[16] Townsend MJ. Molecular and cellular heterogeneity in the Rheumatoid Arthritis synovium: clinical correlates of synovitis. Best practice & research Clinical rheumatology. 2014;28(4):539-49.

[17] Humby F, Lewis M, Ramamoorthi N, Hackney JA, Barnes MR, Bombardieri M, et al. Synovial cellular and molecular signatures stratify clinical response to csDMARD therapy and predict radiographic progression in early rheumatoid arthritis patients. Annals of the rheumatic diseases. 2019;78(6):761-72.

[18] Nielsen MA, Lomholt S, Mellemkjaer A, Andersen MN, Buckley CD, Kragstrup TW. Responses to Cytokine Inhibitors Associated with Cellular Composition in Models of Immune-Mediated Inflammatory Arthritis. ACR Open Rheumatol. 2020;2(1):3-10.

[19] Humby F, Durez P, Buch MH, Lewis MJ, Rizvi H, Rivellese F, et al. Rituximab versus tocilizumab in anti-TNF inadequate responder patients with rheumatoid arthritis (R4RA): 16-week outcomes of a stratified, biopsy-driven, multicentre, open-label, phase 4 randomised controlled trial. Lancet. 2021;397(10271):305-17.

[20] Armaka M, Ospelt C, Pasparakis M, Kollias G. The p55TNFR-IKK2-Ripk3 axis orchestrates arthritis by regulating death and inflammatory pathways in synovial fibroblasts. Nature communications. 2018;9(1):618.

[21] Armaka M, Apostolaki M, Jacques P, Kontoyiannis DL, Elewaut D, Kollias G. Mesenchymal cell targeting by TNF as a common pathogenic principle in chronic inflammatory joint and intestinal diseases. The Journal of experimental medicine. 2008;205(2):331-7.

[22] Bottini N, Firestein GS. Duality of fibroblast-like synoviocytes in RA: passive responders and imprinted aggressors. Nature reviews Rheumatology. 2013;9(1):24-33.

[23] Kato M, Ospelt C, Gay RE, Gay S, Klein K. Dual role of autophagy in stress-induced cell death in rheumatoid arthritis synovial fibroblasts. Arthritis & rheumatology (Hoboken, NJ). 2014;66(1):40-8.

[24] Shin YJ, Han SH, Kim DS, Lee GH, Yoo WH, Kang YM, et al. Autophagy induction and CHOP under-expression promotes survival of fibroblasts from rheumatoid arthritis patients under endoplasmic reticulum stress. Arthritis research & therapy. 2010;12(1):R19.

[25] Matsumoto S, Müller-Ladner U, Gay RE, Nishioka K, Gay S. Ultrastructural demonstration of apoptosis, Fas and Bcl-2 expression of rheumatoid synovial fibroblasts. The Journal of rheumatology. 1996;23(8):1345-52.

[26] Marinova-Mutafchieva L, Williams RO, Funa K, Maini RN, Zvaifler NJ. Inflammation is preceded by tumor necrosis factor-dependent infiltration of mesenchymal cells in experimental arthritis. Arthritis and rheumatism. 2002;46(2):507-13.

[27] Roelofs AJ, Zupan J, Riemen AHK, Kania K, Ansboro S, White N, et al. Joint morphogenetic cells in the adult mammalian synovium. Nature communications. 2017;8:15040.

[28] Smith RS, Smith TJ, Blieden TM, Phipps RP. Fibroblasts as sentinel cells. Synthesis of chemokines and regulation of inflammation. The American journal of pathology. 1997;151(2):317-22.

[29] Salmon M, Scheel-Toellner D, Huissoon AP, Pilling D, Shamsadeen N, Hyde H, et al. Inhibition of T cell apoptosis in the rheumatoid synovium. The Journal of clinical investigation. 1997;99(3):439-46.

[30] Filer A, Parsonage G, Smith E, Osborne C, Thomas AM, Curnow SJ, et al. Differential survival of leukocyte subsets mediated by synovial, bone marrow, and skin fibroblasts: site-specific versus activation-dependent survival of T cells and neutrophils. Arthritis and rheumatism. 2006;54(7):2096-108.

[31] Buckley CD, Pilling D, Lord JM, Akbar AN, Scheel-Toellner D, Salmon M. Fibroblasts regulate the switch from acute resolving to chronic persistent inflammation. Trends Immunol. 2001;22(4):199-204.

[32] Fox DA, Gizinski A, Morgan R, Lundy SK. Cell-cell interactions in

rheumatoid arthritis synovium. Rheumatic diseases clinics of North America. 2010;36(2):311-23.

[33] Kyburz D, Rethage J, Seibl R, Lauener R, Gay RE, Carson DA, et al. Bacterial peptidoglycans but not CpG oligodeoxynucleotides activate synovial fibroblasts by toll-like receptor signaling. Arthritis and rheumatism. 2003;48(3):642-50.

[34] Tran CN, Davis MJ, Tesmer LA, Endres JL, Motyl CD, Smuda C, et al. Presentation of arthritogenic peptide to antigen-specific T cells by fibroblast-like synoviocytes. Arthritis and rheumatism. 2007;56(5):1497-506.

[35] Barone F, Gardner DH, Nayar S, Steinthal N, Buckley CD, Luther SA. Stromal Fibroblasts in Tertiary Lymphoid Structures: A Novel Target in Chronic Inflammation. Front Immunol. 2016;7:477.

[36] Hamann J, Wishaupt JO, van Lier RA, Smeets TJ, Breedveld FC, Tak PP. Expression of the activation antigen CD97 and its ligand CD55 in rheumatoid synovial tissue. Arthritis and rheumatism. 1999;42(4):650-8.

[37] Müller-Ladner U, Ospelt C, Gay S, Distler O, Pap T. Cells of the synovium in rheumatoid arthritis. Synovial fibroblasts. Arthritis research & therapy. 2007;9(6):223.

[38] Kiener HP, Niederreiter B, Lee DM, Jimenez-Boj E, Smolen JS, Brenner MB. Cadherin 11 promotes invasive behavior of fibroblast-like synoviocytes. Arthritis and rheumatism. 2009;60(5):1305-10.

[39] Udalova IA, Mantovani A, Feldmann M. Macrophage heterogeneity in the context of rheumatoid arthritis. Nature reviews Rheumatology. 2016;12(8):472-85.

[40] Mulherin D, Fitzgerald O, Bresnihan B. Synovial tissue macrophage populations and articular damage in rheumatoid arthritis. Arthritis and rheumatism. 1996;39(1):115-24.

[41] Salisbury AK, Duke O, Poulter LW. Macrophage-like cells of the pannus area in rheumatoid arthritic joints. Scand J Rheumatol. 1987;16(4):263-72.

[42] Chong SG, Sato S, Kolb M, Gauldie J. Fibrocytes and fibroblasts-Where are we now. The international journal of biochemistry & cell biology. 2019;116:105595.

[43] Stephenson W, Donlin LT, Butler A, Rozo C, Bracken B, Rashidfarrokhi A, et al. Single-cell RNA-seq of rheumatoid arthritis synovial tissue using low-cost microfluidic instrumentation. Nature communications. 2018;9(1):791.

[44] Mizoguchi F, Slowikowski K, Wei K, Marshall JL, Rao DA, Chang SK, et al. Functionally distinct disease-associated fibroblast subsets in rheumatoid arthritis. Nature communications. 2018;9(1):789.

[45] Croft AP, Campos J, Jansen K, Turner JD, Marshall J, Attar M, et al. Distinct fibroblast subsets drive inflammation and damage in arthritis. Nature. 2019;570(7760):246-51.

[46] Orange DE, Yao V, Sawicka K, Fak J, Frank MO, Parveen S, et al. RNA Identification of PRIME Cells Predicting Rheumatoid Arthritis Flares. The New England journal of medicine. 2020;383(3):218-28.

[47] Manzo A, Bugatti S, Caporali R, Prevo R, Jackson DG, Uguccioni M, et al. CCL21 expression pattern of human secondary lymphoid organ stroma is conserved in inflammatory lesions with lymphoid neogenesis. The American journal of pathology. 2007;171(5): 1549-62.

[48] Manzo A, Paoletti S, Carulli M, Blades MC, Barone F, Yanni G, et al.

Systematic microanatomical analysis of CXCL13 and CCL21 in situ production and progressive lymphoid organization in rheumatoid synovitis. Eur J Immunol. 2005;35(5):1347-59.

[49] Mueller CG, Hess E. Emerging Functions of RANKL in Lymphoid Tissues. Front Immunol. 2012;3:261.

[50] Caulfield JP, Hein A, Dynesius-Trentham R, Trentham DE. Morphologic demonstration of two stages in the development of type II collagen-induced arthritis. Lab Invest. 1982;46(3):321-43.

[51] Lefèvre S, Knedla A, Tennie C, Kampmann A, Wunrau C, Dinser R, et al. Synovial fibroblasts spread rheumatoid arthritis to unaffected joints. Nature medicine. 2009;15(12):1414-20.

[52] Müller-Ladner U, Kriegsmann J, Franklin BN, Matsumoto S, Geiler T, Gay RE, et al. Synovial fibroblasts of patients with rheumatoid arthritis attach to and invade normal human cartilage when engrafted into SCID mice. The American journal of pathology. 1996;149(5):1607-15.

[53] Janssens R, Struyf S, Proost P. Pathological roles of the homeostatic chemokine CXCL12. Cytokine Growth Factor Rev. 2018;44:51-68.

[54] Allis CD, Jenuwein T. The molecular hallmarks of epigenetic control. Nat Rev Genet. 2016;17(8):487-500.

[55] Frank-Bertoncelj M, Trenkmann M, Klein K, Karouzakis E, Rehrauer H, Bratus A, et al. Epigenetically-driven anatomical diversity of synovial fibroblasts guides joint-specific fibroblast functions. Nature communications. 2017;8:14852.

[56] Pap T, Nawrath M, Heinrich J, Bosse M, Baier A, Hummel KM, et al. Cooperation of Ras- and c-Myc-dependent pathways in regulating the growth and invasiveness of synovial fibroblasts in rheumatoid arthritis. Arthritis and rheumatism. 2004;50(9):2794-802.

[57] Pap T, Aupperle KR, Gay S, Firestein GS, Gay RE. Invasiveness of synovial fibroblasts is regulated by p53 in the SCID mouse in vivo model of cartilage invasion. Arthritis and rheumatism. 2001;44(3):676-81.

[58] Miagkov AV, Kovalenko DV, Brown CE, Didsbury JR, Cogswell JP, Stimpson SA, et al. NF-kappaB activation provides the potential link between inflammation and hyperplasia in the arthritic joint. Proceedings of the National Academy of Sciences of the United States of America. 1998;95(23):13859-64.

[59] Ahn JK, Kim S, Hwang J, Kim J, Kim KH, Cha HS. GC/TOF-MS-based metabolomic profiling in cultured fibroblast-like synoviocytes from rheumatoid arthritis. Joint, bone, spine : revue du rhumatisme. 2016;83(6): 707-13.

[60] Friščić J, Böttcher M, Reinwald C, Bruns H, Wirth B, Popp S-J, et al. The complement system drives local inflammatory tissue priming by metabolic reprogramming of synovial fibroblasts. Immunity. 2021.

[61] Alivernini S, MacDonald L, Elmesmari A, Finlay S, Tolusso B, Gigante MR, et al. Distinct synovial tissue macrophage subsets regulate inflammation and remission in rheumatoid arthritis. Nature medicine. 2020;26(8):1295-306.

[62] Bromley M, Woolley DE. Histopathology of the rheumatoid lesion. Identification of cell types at sites of cartilage erosion. Arthritis and rheumatism. 1984;27(8):857-63.

[63] Fassbender HG. Histomorphological basis of articular cartilage destruction in

rheumatoid arthritis. Coll Relat Res. 1983;3(2):141-55.

[64] Tolboom TC, Pieterman E, van der Laan WH, Toes RE, Huidekoper AL, Nelissen RG, et al. Invasive properties of fibroblast-like synoviocytes: correlation with growth characteristics and expression of MMP-1, MMP-3, and MMP-10. Annals of the rheumatic diseases. 2002;61(11):975-80.

[65] Wäldele S, Koers-Wunrau C, Beckmann D, Korb-Pap A, Wehmeyer C, Pap T, et al. Deficiency of fibroblast activation protein alpha ameliorates cartilage destruction in inflammatory destructive arthritis. Arthritis research & therapy. 2015;17(1):12.

[66] Sun M, Rethi B, Krishnamurthy A, Joshua V, Circiumaru A, Hensvold AH, et al. Anticitrullinated protein antibodies facilitate migration of synovial tissue-derived fibroblasts. Annals of the rheumatic diseases. 2019;78(12):1621-31.

[67] Tolboom TC, van der Helm-Van Mil AH, Nelissen RG, Breedveld FC, Toes RE, Huizinga TW. Invasiveness of fibroblast-like synoviocytes is an individual patient characteristic associated with the rate of joint destruction in patients with rheumatoid arthritis. Arthritis and rheumatism. 2005;52(7):1999-2002.

[68] Pettit AR, Walsh NC, Manning C, Goldring SR, Gravallese EM. RANKL protein is expressed at the pannus-bone interface at sites of articular bone erosion in rheumatoid arthritis. Rheumatology. 2006;45(9):1068-76.

[69] Diarra D, Stolina M, Polzer K, Zwerina J, Ominsky MS, Dwyer D, et al. Dickkopf-1 is a master regulator of joint remodeling. Nature medicine. 2007;13(2):156-63.

[70] Siiskonen H, Oikari S, Pasonen-Seppänen S, Rilla K. Hyaluronan synthase 1: a mysterious enzyme with unexpected functions. Front Immunol. 2015;6:43.

[71] Dho SH, Lim JC, Kim LK. Beyond the Role of CD55 as a Complement Component. Immune Netw. 2018;18(1):e11.

[72] Choi IY, Karpus ON, Turner JD, Hardie D, Marshall JL, de Hair MJH, et al. Stromal cell markers are differentially expressed in the synovial tissue of patients with early arthritis. PloS one. 2017;12(8):e0182751.

[73] Karpus ON, Kiener HP, Niederreiter B, Yilmaz-Elis AS, van der Kaa J, Ramaglia V, et al. CD55 deposited on synovial collagen fibers protects from immune complex-mediated arthritis. Arthritis research & therapy. 2015;17(1):6.

[74] Das N, Schmidt TA, Krawetz RJ, Dufour A. Proteoglycan 4: From Mere Lubricant to Regulator of Tissue Homeostasis and Inflammation: Does proteoglycan 4 have the ability to buffer the inflammatory response? Bioessays. 2019;41(1):e1800166.

[75] Gururaja Rao S, Patel NJ, Singh H. Intracellular Chloride Channels: Novel Biomarkers in Diseases. Front Physiol. 2020;11:96.

[76] Taylor SR, Markesbery MG, Harding PA. Heparin-binding epidermal growth factor-like growth factor (HB-EGF) and proteolytic processing by a disintegrin and metalloproteinases (ADAM): a regulator of several pathways. Semin Cell Dev Biol. 2014;28:22-30.

[77] Kuo D, Ding J, Cohn IS, Zhang F, Wei K, Rao DA, et al. HBEGF(+) macrophages in rheumatoid arthritis induce fibroblast invasiveness. Sci Transl Med. 2019;11(491).

[78] Leyton L, Díaz J, Martínez S, Palacios E, Pérez LA, Pérez RD.

Thy-1/CD90 a Bidirectional and Lateral Signaling Scaffold. Front Cell Dev Biol. 2019;7:132.

[79] Sidney LE, Branch MJ, Dunphy SE, Dua HS, Hopkinson A. Concise review: evidence for CD34 as a common marker for diverse progenitors. Stem cells. 2014;32(6):1380-9.

[80] Bowness P. HLA-B27. Annual review of immunology. 2015;33:29-48.

[81] Kurkó J, Besenyei T, Laki J, Glant TT, Mikecz K, Szekanecz Z. Genetics of rheumatoid arthritis - a comprehensive review. Clin Rev Allergy Immunol. 2013;45(2):170-9.

[82] Niehrs C. Function and biological roles of the Dickkopf family of Wnt modulators. Oncogene. 2006;25(57):7469-81.

[83] Snelling SJ, Davidson RK, Swingler TE, Le LT, Barter MJ, Culley KL, et al. Dickkopf-3 is upregulated in osteoarthritis and has a chondroprotective role. Osteoarthritis and cartilage / OARS, Osteoarthritis Research Society. 2016;24(5):883-91.

[84] Ludwig J, Federico G, Prokosch S, Küblbeck G, Schmitt S, Klevenz A, et al. Dickkopf-3 acts as a modulator of B cell fate and function. Journal of immunology. 2015;194(6):2624-34.

[85] Papatriantafyllou M, Moldenhauer G, Ludwig J, Tafuri A, Garbi N, Hollmann G, et al. Dickkopf-3, an immune modulator in peripheral CD8 T-cell tolerance. Proceedings of the National Academy of Sciences of the United States of America. 2012;109(5):1631-6.

[86] Itonaga I, Fujikawa Y, Sabokbar A, Murray DW, Athanasou NA. Rheumatoid arthritis synovial macrophage-osteoclast differentiation is osteoprotegerin ligand-dependent. J Pathol. 2000;192(1):97-104.

[87] Starup-Linde J, Viggers R, Handberg A. Osteoglycin and Bone-a Systematic Review. Current osteoporosis reports. 2019;17(5):250-5.

[88] Bonelli M, Dalwigk K, Platzer A, Olmos Calvo I, Hayer S, Niederreiter B, et al. IRF1 is critical for the TNF-driven interferon response in rheumatoid fibroblast-like synoviocytes : JAKinibs suppress the interferon response in RA-FLSs. Experimental & molecular medicine. 2019;51(7):75.

[89] Maruyama K, Muramatsu H, Ishiguro N, Muramatsu T. Midkine, a heparin-binding growth factor, is fundamentally involved in the pathogenesis of rheumatoid arthritis. Arthritis and rheumatism. 2004;50(5):1420-9.

[90] Neumann E, Barnum SR, Tarner IH, Echols J, Fleck M, Judex M, et al. Local production of complement proteins in rheumatoid arthritis synovium. Arthritis and rheumatism. 2002;46(4):934-45.

[91] Sawada Y, Mashima E, Saito-Sasaki N, Nakamura M. The Role of Cell Adhesion Molecule 1 (CADM1) in Cutaneous Malignancies. International journal of molecular sciences. 2020;21(24).

[92] van der Geest T, Laverman P, Gerrits D, Walgreen B, Helsen MM, Klein C, et al. Liposomal Treatment of Experimental Arthritis Can Be Monitored Noninvasively with a Radiolabeled Anti-Fibroblast Activation Protein Antibody. Journal of nuclear medicine : official publication, Society of Nuclear Medicine. 2017;58(1):151-5.

[93] van der Geest T, Roeleveld DM, Walgreen B, Helsen MM, Nayak TK, Klein C, et al. Imaging fibroblast activation protein to monitor therapeutic effects of neutralizing interleukin-22 in collagen-induced

arthritis. Rheumatology. 2018;57(4):737-47.

[94] Cunningham C AS, Wade S, Low C, Mullan R, Veale D, Fearon U. Characterisation of Rheumatoid and Psoriatic Arthritis Synovial Fibroblasts [abstract]. Arthritis & rheumatology (Hoboken, NJ). 2020;72.

[95] Stebulis JA, Rossetti RG, Atez FJ, Zurier RB. Fibroblast-like synovial cells derived from synovial fluid. The Journal of rheumatology. 2005;32(2):301-6.

[96] Ahn JK, Kim H, Lee J, Bae EK, Cha HS, Koh EM. Phenotypic characterization and invasive properties of synovial fluid-derived adherent cells in rheumatoid arthritis. Inflammation. 2008;31(6):365-71.

[97] Orr C, Vieira-Sousa E, Boyle DL, Buch MH, Buckley CD, Cañete JD, et al. Synovial tissue research: a state-of-the-art review. Nature reviews Rheumatology. 2017;13(8):463-75.

[98] Gerlag DM, Tak PP. How to perform and analyse synovial biopsies. Best practice & research Clinical rheumatology. 2013;27(2):195-207.

[99] Kelly S, Humby F, Filer A, Ng N, Di Cicco M, Hands RE, et al. Ultrasound-guided synovial biopsy: a safe, well-tolerated and reliable technique for obtaining high-quality synovial tissue from both large and small joints in early arthritis patients. Annals of the rheumatic diseases. 2015;74(3):611-7.

[100] Lazarou I, D'Agostino MA, Naredo E, Humby F, Filer A, Kelly SG. Ultrasound-guided synovial biopsy: a systematic review according to the OMERACT filter and recommendations for minimal reporting standards in clinical studies. Rheumatology. 2015;54(10):1867-75.

[101] Svensson MND, Zoccheddu M, Yang S, Nygaard G, Secchi C, Doody KM, et al. Synoviocyte-targeted therapy synergizes with TNF inhibition in arthritis reversal. Sci Adv. 2020;6(26):eaba4353.

[102] Stougaard J, Lomholt S, Ommen P, Kelsen J, Kragstrup TW. The antifibrotic drug pirfenidone inhibits spondyloarthritis fibroblast-like synoviocytes and osteoblasts in vitro. BMC Rheumatology. 2018;2(1):33.

[103] Siebert S, Pratt AG, Stocken DD, Morton M, Cranston A, Cole M, et al. Targeting the rheumatoid arthritis synovial fibroblast via cyclin dependent kinase inhibition: An early phase trial. Medicine (Baltimore). 2020;99(26):e20458.

[104] Brennen WN, DL JT, Jiang W, Krueger TE, Antony L, Denmeade SR, et al. Overcoming stromal barriers to immuno-oncological responses via fibroblast activation protein-targeted therapy. Immunotherapy. 2021;13(2):155-75.

[105] Xu T, Zhao Y, Ding H, Cai L, Zhou Z, Song Z, et al. [(68)Ga] Ga-DOTA-FAPI-04 PET/CT imaging in a case of prostate cancer with shoulder arthritis. European journal of nuclear medicine and molecular imaging. 2020.

[106] Montero-Melendez T, Nagano A, Chelala C, Filer A, Buckley CD, Perretti M. Therapeutic senescence via GPCR activation in synovial fibroblasts facilitates resolution of arthritis. Nature communications. 2020;11(1):745.

[107] Wei K, Korsunsky I, Marshall JL, Gao A, Watts GFM, Major T, et al. Notch signalling drives synovial fibroblast identity and arthritis pathology. Nature. 2020;582(7811):259-64.

[108] Kragstrup TW, Sohn DH, Lepus CM, Onuma K, Wang Q, Robinson WH, et al. Fibroblast-like synovial cell production of extra domain A fibronectin associates with

inflammation in osteoarthritis. BMC Rheumatol. 2019;3:46.

[109] Kriegsmann J, Berndt A, Hansen T, Borsi L, Zardi L, Bräuer R, et al. Expression of fibronectin splice variants and oncofetal glycosylated fibronectin in the synovial membranes of patients with rheumatoid arthritis and osteoarthritis. Rheumatology international. 2004;24(1):25-33.

[110] Kumra H, Reinhardt DP. Fibronectin-targeted drug delivery in cancer. Advanced drug delivery reviews. 2016;97:101-10.

[111] Nygaard G, Firestein GS. Restoring synovial homeostasis in rheumatoid arthritis by targeting fibroblast-like synoviocytes. Nature reviews Rheumatology. 2020;16(6):316-33.

Chapter 6

Fibroblasts in Sjögren's Syndrome

Kerstin Klein

Abstract

The Sjögren's syndrome is an autoimmune disease characterized by chronic inflammation of the exocrine glands, leading to dryness of mucosal surfaces, and often to severe systemic manifestations. Here, the immunomodulatory function of fibroblasts derived from salivary glands, a primary site affected by the Sjögren's syndrome, is discussed. Specific subsets of these fibroblasts drive the formation of tertiary lymphoid structures, which are associated with severe disease and which constitute a risk factor for the development of lymphoma in Sjögren's syndrome. Single cell RNA-sequencing has provided new insights into subsets of fibroblasts in inflamed salivary glands and has provided evidence for the existence of shared inflammation-associated fibroblasts across chronically inflamed tissues. These findings support the concept of targeting the fibroblast compartment in Sjögren's syndrome and other chronic inflammatory diseases. In addition to the immunomodulatory role of fibroblasts, the interaction of the epithelium with fibroblasts is essential for salivary gland homeostasis. Fibroblasts provide essential signals for the regeneration of salivary gland epithelial cells, which is disturbed in Sjögren's syndrome, and leading to the loss of saliva secreting cells and subsequent hyposalivation.

Keywords: Sjögren's syndrome, autoimmunity, inflammation, tertiary lymphoid structure, salivary gland

1. Introduction

1.1 Sjögren's syndrome

The Sjögren's Syndrome (SjS) is a systemic autoimmune disease, most commonly presenting between the fourth and six decades of life. It affects predominantly women, with an estimated female to male ratio of 9:1 [1]. With a prevalence of 0.3 to 1 per 1000 people [1], the SjS represents the second most common rheumatic autoimmune condition after rheumatoid arthritis (RA). The SjS can either occur as single disease, often termed as primary SjS, or is associated with other autoimmune diseases, such as RA, systemic lupus erythematosus (SLE), systemic sclerosis (SSc), or dermatomyositis [2]. Up to now, no disease modifying therapies for SjS have been approved and treatment is mainly symptomatic [3].

The hallmark of SjS is a hypofunction of exocrine glands, in particular salivary and lacrimal glands [3]. Dryness of mouth (xerostomia) and eyes (xerophthalmia), alongside fatigue and pain are the major symptoms affecting more than 80% of patients with SjS [2]. The majority of patients with SjS present with glandular symptoms, which are often present over many years before diagnosis [4]. Whilst often considered as "benign features", these symptoms underpin great patient-reported disability. Other signs of systemic dryness, with scant information regarding the etiology and affecting patients' quality of life, involve the skin, the nose, the throat, the trachea and the vagina [5].

A major classification criterion for SjS is the infiltration of salivary glands with lymphocytes (focus score ≥1, in minor labial salivary gland biopsy), a condition called sialadenitis. The second major classification criterion is the presence of anti-SSA/Ro auto-antibodies, which is mandatory in patients with a lack of sialadenitis [3]. In 30 to 40% of patients, systemic epithelial and extra-epithelial manifestations occur that can affect the joints, skin, lungs, kidneys and nervous system [2].

People with SjS have increased morbidity and mortality compared to the general population [4]. Although being a rare event, the risk of B-cell lymphomas is 15 to 20 times higher in patients with SjS as the general population and accounts for the leading cause with an impact on patients's survival [2, 4]. The most common type of lymphomas in patients with SjS are mucosa-associated lymphoid tissue (MALT) lymphomas. Chronic activation of B cells at the primary sites affected by SjS, such as the salivary glands, was attributed to the development of lymphoma. Several risk factors have been defined for the development of lymphoma in patients with SjS; among them is the presence of ectopic germinal centers in tertiary lymphoid structures (TLS) [2].

1.2 Epithelial cell activation is central in the pathogenesis in SjS

The SjS develops in genetically predisposed individuals upon exposure to stress factors. Hormones as well as infectious agents, and in particular viruses, are assumed to play key roles in the pathogenesis of the SjS. Activated epithelial cells in salivary glands are the central cell type in the current concept underlying the pathogenesis. They are on the one hand drivers of the ongoing inflammation and on the other hand, due to the excess of apoptosis of epithelial cells in salivary glands, a source of auto-antigens for infiltrating lymphocytes [6]. Epithelial cells respond to and produce pro-inflammatory cytokines and chemokines and thus, promote inflammation. They produce MHC-II and co-stimulatory molecules, enabling them to directly interact with and activate T-cells. Furthermore, they produce B-cell activating factor (BAFF), inducing the activation and survival of B cells [7]. Many of these characteristics have been previously described for fibroblasts, e.g. in the synovium of rheumatoid arthritis patients, and analogies of synovial fibroblasts with salivary gland-derived fibroblasts have been recognized [7, 8]. However, the ability of salivary gland-derived fibroblasts to exert similar functions is only at the beginning to be characterized in detail.

2. Fibroblasts in tertiary lymphoid structures

2.1 Tertiary lymphoid structures are often present in autoimmune diseases

TLS, or ectopic lymphoid organs (ELS), often develop at sites of inflammation in target tissues. Their formation has been associated with chronic inflammation, autoimmune disease, cancer, and transplant rejection [9]. TLS are sites of ectopic auto-antibody production and expansion of potential autoreactive B cell clones [7, 10]. The formation of TLS in salivary glands is an established model for studying TLS formation in autoimmunity in general. The frequency of the presence of TLS varies among different autoimmune diseases, with a high frequency in autoimmune thyroiditis and low presence in systemic lupus erythematosus [10]. Approximately 30–40% of patients with SjS exhibit TLS in their salivary glands, the primary sites of the disease [11, 12].

A similar percentage of TLS is found in patients with rheumatoid arthritis, in which TLS are associated with a lympho-myeloid pathotype that represents a distinct disease entity as the diffuse myeloid and pauci-immune fibroid pathotpyes [13]. Hence, the presence and absence of TLS in salivary glands of patients with SjS might underlie different pathophysiological processes in different, not yet characterized, disease subsets. The formation of TLS is across autoimmune diseases associated with more severe disease and poor prognosis [7].

TLS often share several typical structural characteristics with secondary lymphoid tissues (lymph nodes, tonsils, spleen, Peyer's patches, mucosa-associated lymphoid tissues), including highly organized lymphocytic aggregates, with T and B cell segregation, the development of high endothelial venules, and follicular dendritic cell networks. In contrast to secondary lymphoid tissues, the lymphocytic aggregates found in TLS can range from a simple aggregates to highly ordered structures with bona fide germinal centers that support the production of autoreactive plasma cells [9, 10]. TLS formation and secondary lymphoid tissue development follow numerous overlapping signaling pathways, however, the cellular sources of signaling molecules differ [10]. In contrast to secondary lymphoid structures whose development is initiated at the embryonic stage, TLS develop postnatally in response to inflammatory signals, where they provide a specialized pro-inflammatory environment that plays a key role in perpetuating disease progression in autoimmune conditions [7, 14]. Podoplanin (pdpn)-expressing fibroblastic reticular cells in secondary lymphoid organs and pdpn$^+$ stromal fibroblasts in TLS provide signals and the scaffold structure that foster the interaction of T cells with dendritic cells, and hence drive innate and adaptive immune responses [15, 16].

2.2 Tertiary lymphoid structures are associated with severe disease in Sjögren's syndrome

The routine histopathological examination of minor salivary gland biopsies carries a substantial prognostic value regarding disease severity and outcome [17]. Higher inflammatory scores, and the presence of germinal center-like structures in particular, in salivary glands of patients with SjS were associated with more severe disease, illustrated by elevated titers of rheumatoid factor, anti-Ro/SSA and anti-Ro/SSB auto-antibodies, enhanced levels of local and systemic pro-inflammatory mediators and a reduced saliva secretion [11, 17, 18]. Germinal center-like structures have been identified in approximately 25% of patients with SjS [17, 19]. Their presence at time of diagnosis, or sole high lymphocytic scores, were shown to account as independent risk factors for the development of Non-Hodgkin's lymphomas in patients with SjS [17, 19].

Given the pivotal role of TLS in SjS, the identification of factors and pathological mechanisms triggering and regulating their formation and those of germinal center-like structures is of high interest in order to identify potential targets for drug development.

2.3 Adenoviral infection using retrograde excretory duct cannulation is a model of SjS

Studying the chronology of TLS formation and associated cell types in animal models, together with complementary evaluation of human salivary gland specimens, provided new insights into pathomechanisms associated with sialadenitis in SjS, and unraveled the analogy of TLS formation to the development of secondary lymphoid organs. A model that proved to be of particular value for studying salivary gland inflammation in SjS, and the formation of TLS in autoimmune processes in general, is the selective submandibular gland administration of a replication-defective adenovirus 5 (AdV5) through retrograde excretory duct cannulation in wild-type C57/Bl76 mice. These mice were shown to resemble several hallmarks of SjS, including lymphocytic infiltration of salivary glands, TLS formation, anti-nuclear autoantibody (ANA) formation, and reduction in salivary flow indicative of excretory gland dysfunction [20]. Cannulated mice developed SjS-like periductal lymphoid aggregates within two weeks after AdV5 delivery. Within three weeks, the inducible TLS acquired progressively hallmarks of functional germinal centers, with segregated B and T cell areas, high endothelial venules in T-cell rich areas, and follicular dendritic cell networks in up to 70% of the lymphocytic aggregates. Local expression of activation-induced cytidine deaminase (AID), the enzyme required for Ig somatic hypermutation and class-switch recombination, pointed to the functional activation of B cells in TLS [20].

2.4 Fibroblasts drive the formation of tertiary lymphoid structures

During secondary lymphoid organ development in embryogenesis, mesenchymal precursor cell maturate into intercellular adhesion molecule-1 (ICAM-1)^{high}, vascular cell adhesion molecule-1 (VCAM-1)^{high} organizer cells, in a process that is dependent on lymphoid tissue inducer cells and lymphotoxin β receptor (LTβR) signaling. This leads to a sustained stromal cell production of interleukin 7 (IL7), C-X-C motif chemokine ligand 13 (CXCL13) and to a lesser extent C-C motif chemokine ligand 21 (CCL21) [21]. The subsequent migration of lymphocytes into the anlagen is responsible for the full differentiation of fibroblastic reticular cells within distinct areas of the secondary lymphoid organ [22–24].

In TLS of salivary glands of patients with SjS, a network of pdpn^{+} and fibroblast activating protein (FAP)$^{+}$ fibroblasts were identified that support the formation of TLS [24]. The same markers have been previously identified on fibroblast reticular cells in lymph nodes [15, 25], which provide, by the secretion of CCL19 and CCL21, the key factors for the migration and retention of T cells in secondary lymphoid organs [16, 25, 26]. Among the pdpn^{+} fibroblasts in TLS, two functionally distinct populations have been identified in human salivary glands that provide the signals for lymphocyte survival and organization within TLS, respectively (**Figure 1**) [24]. The first cluster of pdpn^{+} fibroblasts, was characterized by high expression of FAP, ICAM-1, VCAM-1 and CD34 [24]. Pdpn+CD34+ fibroblasts in TLS produced IL7 and BAFF, underlying their function in supporting lymphocyte survival and homeostasis [24]. The second cluster of pdpn^{+} CD34^{-} fibroblasts was characterized by high expression levels of CXCL13, CCL19 and CCL21. Expansion of a similar network of pdpn+ fibroblasts has been observed upon salivary gland infection of mice with Ad5V. Of note, this expansion occurred before lymphocyte infiltration, suggesting a pivotal, early role for fibroblasts in SjS. Fibroblasts in TLS of cannulated mouse salivary glands expressed CXCL13, CCL19, BAFF, IL7 and LTβR, with an increased expression of lymphoid chemokines specifically in the ICAM-1^{+} VCAM-1^{+} subpopulation of pdpn^{+} fibroblasts [24].

2.5 IL13 and IL22 induce the formation of tertiary lymphoid structures

Pdnp+ fibroblasts in human TLS expressed receptors for and responded to stimulation with IL13, IL4, IL22, TNF, and LTα1β2 [24, 27]. Elevated levels of IL13 have been detected in serum of patients with SjS, where they correlated with titers of anti-Ro/SSA auto-antibodies [28], and in Id3 knockout mice, a model for T cell mediated SjS [29, 30]. Also, high levels of IL22 in sera of patients with SjS have been shown to correlate with clinically relevant parameters, such as reduced salivary

DOI: http://dx.doi.org/10.5772/intechopen.98946

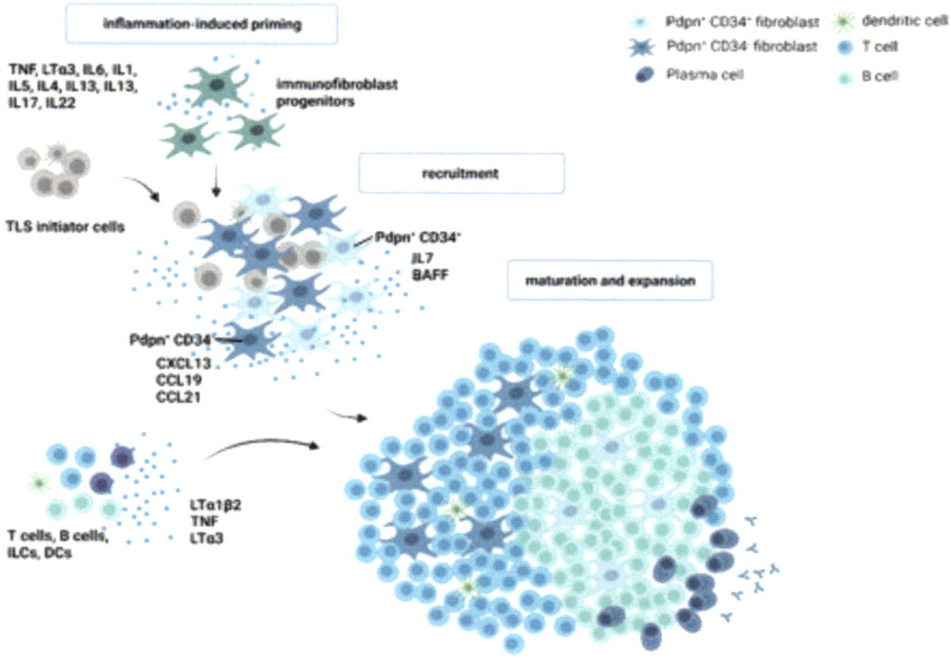

Figure 1.
Stromal fibroblast populations contribute to the formation of tertiary lymphoid structures (TLS). Created by BioRender.com. DCs, dendritic cells; ILCs, innate lymphoid cells.

flow, hypergammaglobulinemia, as well as serum titers of rheumatoid factor, anti-Ro/SSA and anti-Ro/SSB auto-antibodies [31]. Together these data suggested a potential link between increased levels of IL13 and IL22 with the auto-antibody production in SjS.

IL13 stimulation of cultured human salivary gland fibroblasts, in synergy with TNF and LTα1β2, induced the expression of VCAM-1, ICAM-1 and pdpn *in vitro* (**Table 1**). This function was confirmed *in vivo*. Innate lymphoid cells, fibroblasts and epithelial cells have been identified as the source of IL-13 in the developing TLS. IL13 expression was induced rapidly within a few hours upon AdV5 administration in mice, leading to the priming of immunofibroblast progenitors by activation of IL4 receptor signaling, and the subsequent expression of pdpn, ICAM-1 and VCAM-1. AdV5 administration in $IL4R^{-/-}$ mice led to a disturbed TLS assembly, and salivary glands were characterized by reduced expression levels of CXCL13 and CCL21, smaller inflammatory foci and an abolished autoantibody production. The early priming of immunofibroblasts by IL13 was independent of the presence of lymphocytes [24].

In contrast to IL13, IL-22 stimulation of cultured human salivary gland fibroblasts induced proliferation but did not induce the expression of pdpn, ICAM-1 and VCAM-1 *in vitro* [24]. Studies in cannulated mice revealed that the induction of IL22 was, similarly to the induction of IL13, an early event after AdV5 delivery in TLS formation. The main sources of IL22 in the developing TLS were T cells, along with innate lymphoid cells and natural killer cells. IL22 induced the expression of CXCL13 in stromal fibroblasts and the expression of CXCL12 in epithelial cells, leading to the subsequent B cell aggregation and auto-antibody production [27]. Together these data demonstrated that IL13 mediates the early priming of fibroblasts in the developing TLS, and IL22 is responsible for the expansion of the fibroblastic network. These early steps in TLS development were independent of

Chemokines	Producing cells	Receptor	Function on target cells
IL13	Innate lymphoid cells Fibroblasts Epithelial cells	IL4R	Fibroblast priming, induces expression of pdpn, VCAM1-, ICAM-1
IL22	T cells Innate lymphoid cells Natural killer cells	IL22Rα	Proliferation of fibroblasts, expansion of the fibroblast network
LTα1β2	Lymphoid tissue inducer cells	LTβR	Final differentiation of fibroblasts in lymphoid structures
CXCL19	Fibroblasts	CXCR7	T cells and dendritic cells chemotaxis
CXCL21	Fibroblasts	CXCR7	Natural killer cells, dendritic cells, T cells chemotaxis
CXCL12	Epithelial cells	CXCR4	Lymphocyte retention inside the lymphoid structures
CXCL13	Fibroblasts	CXCR5	B cells, T cells chemotaxis
BAFF	Fibroblasts Epithelial cells	BAFFR	B cell activation and survival

Table 1.
Chemokines involved in the formation of tertiary lymphoid structures in salivary glands of patients with Sjögren's syndrome.

LTα1β2 and RORγ^{+} lymphoid tissue inducer cells [24], which regulate the final maturation of fibroblastic reticular cells in the development of secondary lymphoid organs [21]. However, studies in LTβr$^{-/-}$ and RORγ$^{-/-}$ mice have underlined their critical role in the final differentiation and stabilization of the functional phenotype of immunofibroblasts at later stages of the TLS assembly [24].

3. Overlap of fibroblasts from patients with SjS and other inflammatory diseases

3.1 Single cell RNA sequencing identifies fibroblast clusters across diseases

The asset of single cell RNA sequencing (scRNA-seq) technologies has enabled the identification of different fibroblasts populations associated with chronic inflammation across different diseases and anatomical sites [32–39]. Given the pro-inflammatory role of fibroblasts and their ability to carry a certain degree of inflammatory memory [40], interfering with fibroblasts has become a new potential therapeutic strategy in chronic inflammatory diseases.

In a recent study, scRNA-seq data sets derived from four different inflammatory diseases, namely rheumatoid arthritis, interstitial lung disease, ulcerative colitis and the SjS were integrated, with the aim to provide a stromal cell atlas to identify pathogenic fibroblast subsets shared across diseases [8]. For each inflamed tissue, non-inflamed control tissues were included in the analysis. With respect to the SjS, biopsies derived from minor salivary gland biopsies of patients with SjS were compared to those from patients with sicca symptoms, characterized as non-autoimmune dryness, and who did not fulfill the classification criteria for SjS. Given the lack of a universal fibroblast marker, fibroblasts in this study were characterized by the expression of collagen (COL) 1A1 and defined as non-epithelial, non-immune, non-endothelial, and non-mural cells based on the respective specific markers for those cell types. By pooling the scRNA-seq data sets from salivary glands, lungs, the

Cluster	Shared markers	Other markers, localization, and characteristics	Shared function
0	n.d.	SG: n.d. Lung: n.d. Synovium: PRG4⁺ lining SF Gut: WNT5B⁺ villus-associated GF	n.d.
1	n.d.	SG: n.d. Lung: n.d. Synovium: THY1⁺ sublining Gut: WNT2B⁺ crypt-associated GF	n.d.
2	n.d.	SG: n.d. Lung: n.d. Synovium: THY1⁺ sublining Gut: WNT2B⁺ crypt-associated GF	n.d.
3	n.d.	SG: n.d. Lung: n.d. Synovium: THY1⁺ sublining Gut: WNT2B⁺ crypt-associated GF	n.d.
4	SPARC⁺ COL3A1⁺	SG: CD34⁺ Lung: myofibroblasts Synovium: split between DKK3⁺ and THY1⁺ sublining SF, $CD90^{hi}$ NOTCH3-activated, perivascular Gut: split between inflammatory and myofibroblasts	crosstalk with endothelial cells
5	FBLN1⁺	SG: n.d. Lung: HAS1⁺PLIN2⁺ Synovium: CD34⁺THY1⁺ Gut: RSPO3⁺	n.d.
6	n.d.	SG: n.d. Lung: n.d. Synovium: PRG4⁺ lining SF Gut: WNT5B⁺ villus-associated GF	n.d.
7	n.d.	SG: n.d. Lung: n.d. Synovium: n.d. Gut: n.d.	n.d.
8	PTGS2⁺ SEMA4A⁺	SG: n.d. Lung: n.d. Synovium: THY1⁺ sublining Gut: WNT2B⁺ crypt-associated GF	n.d.
9	CD34⁺ MFAP5⁺	SG: n.d. Lung: HAS1⁺PLIN2⁺ Synovium: CD34⁺THY1⁺ Gut: RSPO3⁺	n.d.
10		SG: n.d. Lung: n.d. Synovium: PRG4⁺ lining SF Gut: WNT5B⁺ villus-associated GF	n.d.
11	CXCL10⁺ CCL19⁺	SG: CCL19⁺PDPN⁺ Lung: n.d. Synovium: THY1⁺ sublining, $HLA\text{-}DRA^{hi}$ SF Gut: RSPO3⁺, $WNT2B^{+}Fos^{hi}$	interaction with immune cells
12	n.d.	SG: n.d. Lung: n.d. Synovium: PRG4⁺ lining SF Gut: WNT5B⁺ villus-associated GF	n.d.

Cluster	Shared markers	Other markers, localization, and characteristics	Shared function
13	MYH11$^+$	SG: n.d. Lung: myofibroblasts Synovium: n.d. Gut: myofibroblasts	n.d.

GF, gut fibroblast; n.d., not defined; SF, synovial fibroblast.

Table 2.
Shared fibroblasts clusters between salivary gland (SG), lung, synovium, and gut, as defined by Korsynsky et al. [8].

synovium and the gut, 14 clusters of fibroblasts have been identified, each of them consisting of genes that were shared across different tissues in addition to tissue-specific genes (**Table 2**). Among these clusters, two of them expanded across tissues in inflamed versus respective non-inflamed controls.

3.2 CXCL10$^+$ CCL19$^+$ fibroblasts: Interactors with immune cells

The first of these shared clusters is characterized by the marker genes CXCL10 and CCL19. Based on a gene set enrichment and pathway analysis, CXCL10$^+$ CCL19$^+$ fibroblasts were identified as a subset that potentially directly interacts with immune cells. Among the enriched pathways were "lymphocyte chemotaxis", "antigen presentation", and "positive regulation of T cell proliferation". Furthermore, scRNA-seq data suggested that CXCL10$^+$ CCL19$^+$ fibroblasts respond to key pro-inflammatory cytokines, including interferon (IFN) γ and IFNα, TNF, IL1, and IL1. The responsiveness to IFNγ and IFNα was specific to CXCL10$^+$ CCL19$^+$ fibroblasts [8]. This might be of high relevance in the context of the SjS, given the pronounced role of type I and II interferon signatures detected in SjS, and their association with more severe disease [41, 42]. CXCL10$^+$ CCL19$^+$ fibroblasts functionally resembled the pdpn$^+$ CD34$^-$ CCL19 expressing fibroblasts that have been described to be involved in the formation of TLS in salivary glands of patients with SjS [24].

3.3 SPARC+ COL3A1+ fibroblasts: a vascular-interacting population

The second shared cluster of fibroblasts that was identified to be expanded across inflamed tissues was characterized by the expression of secreted protein acidic and cysteine rich (SPARC) and COL3A1. SPARC$^+$ COL3A1$^+$ fibroblasts resembled a potentially endothelium-driven activated fibroblast state, characterized by the enrichment of pathways associated with extracellular matrix binding and remodeling. In addition, key developmental and morphogen signaling pathways were enriched, including hedgehog, transforming growth factor (TGF) β, WNT, bone morphogenic protein (BMP) and Notch signaling. By comparing these shared human fibroblast clusters to the temporal activation of fibroblast clusters in the mouse model of dextran sulfate sodium (DSS)-induced colitis, the expansion of SPARC$^+$ COL3A1$^+$ fibroblasts was identified as an early event in the inflammatory process, in which vascular remodeling preceded leukocyte infiltration [8].

4. Fibroblasts in the regeneration of salivary gland epithelial cells

A key process in gland development is the epithelial-mesenchymal interaction [43]. The stromal-derived extracellular matrix is essential for the growth, morphogenesis and differentiation of salivary gland tissues [44]. Extracellular matrix remodeling and fibrosis are pathological features found in minor salivary gland biopsies of patients with SjS, that are associated with salivary gland inflammation, reduced stimulated salivary flow but not with age [44–46]. Point mutations in people with hypohidrotic ectodermal dysplasia (HED) lead to a disturbed signaling between the salivary epithelium and mesenchymal fibroblasts, affecting their gland development. Salivary and sweat glands have the same embryonic origin and people with HED present with defects in salivary glands, sweat glands, teeth and hair [47].

Several studies have pointed out that the correlation of salivary flow with the degree of inflammation in salivary glands of patients with SjS is low [48–51], suggesting that other mechanisms than inflammation underlie hyposalivation in SjS. Salivary gland epithelial cells of patients with SjS are more prone to anoikis, a detachment-induced apoptosis, after activation of Toll-like receptor 3 signaling [52]. In healthy salivary glands, salivary gland stem cells reside in ducts of salivary glands and differentiate into saliva secreting acinar cells to maintain homeostasis. In SjS, salivary gland stem cells are fewer in numbers and exhibit an aged phenotype, with a reduced capacity to self-renew and proliferate [53]. This suggests that saliva production in patients with SjS might not be restored solely be the use of anti-inflammatory drugs. In regenerative medicine approaches, the co-culturing of stem cells together with fibroblasts is essential for engineering secreting salivary epithelial cells [54, 55]. Hence, fibroblasts might also be involved in the disturbed regeneration of salivary gland epithelial cells in SjS and are likely to have functions beyond promoting inflammation.

5. The potential role of fibroblasts in extra-glandular manifestations of the SjS

Extra-glandular manifestations are found in 30–40% of patients with SjS, and can be divided into epithelial and extra-epithelial manifestations that can affect the central and peripheral nervous system, the lungs, lymph nodes, kidneys, joints, the skin and the muscles [2, 4]. A role of fibroblasts in extra-glandular manifestations has not been studied yet, maybe due to limited assess of available tissue samples from affected sites.

Articular manifestations, such as arthralgias and synovitis, are the most common extra-glandular manifestations and affect 30–60% of patients with SjS [2, 56]. Arthritis in patients with SjS is often classified as non-erosive [57]. However, recent more sensitive methods such as ultrasound and magnetic resonance imaging (MRI) have detected erosions in more than one third of SjS patients with joint pain and no previous diagnosis of arthritis [57, 58]. In patients with SjS, arthritis most frequently occurs in proximal interphalangeal (PIP) and metacarpophalangeal (MCP) joints and wrists [57], a pattern that is overlapping with the one found in hands of RA patients [59]. Synovial fibroblasts are the major stroma cells of the joint and play a pivotal role in the pathogenesis of rheumatoid arthritis by promoting the ongoing inflammation and cartilage degradation [60]. The existence of shared fibroblast clusters in salivary glands of SjS patients and synovial tissues of rheumatoid arthritis patients, suggests a role of fibroblasts also in articular manifestations of the SjS. However, this potential role of fibroblasts remains to be proven.

6. Conclusions

The Sjögren's syndrome is a chronic inflammatory autoimmune disease with huge unmet needs for patients and clinicians. No therapies for the treatment of the SjS have been approved so far. The pathogenic processes in the exocrine glands have only partially unraveled. Whereas the contribution of salivary gland epithelial cells has been studied in detail, the functional role of fibroblasts in maintaining epithelial cell function, as well as their role in the regulation of the inflammatory process has only recently been recognized. The potential of targeting the fibroblast compartment in salivary glands of patients with SjS has been underscored by studies characterizing their role in the establishment of TLS as well as by scRNA-seq of minor salivary gland tissues. Together these studies pointed to an early, to a large extent lymphocyte-independent, role of fibroblasts in the pathogenesis of the SjS.

Integration of the scRNA-seq data sets across inflamed human tissues, including minor salivary gland tissues from patients with SjS, together with scRNA-seq data sets from mouse models, have suggested a two stage mechanism for fibroblast activation and fibroblast-mediated regulation of inflammation. In this model, the expansion of $SPARC^+$ $COL3A1^+$ vascular-associated fibroblasts initiates vascular remodeling and subsequent leukocyte infiltration and precedes the expansion of $CXCL10^+$ $CCL19^+$ immune-interacting fibroblasts.

$CXCL10^+$ $CCL19^+$ immune-interacting fibroblasts functionally resemble $pdpn^+$ $CD34^-$ CCL19 expressing fibroblasts that are critically involved in TLS assembly. Formation of TLS is initiated after experimental salivary gland infection by IL13 and IL22 that prime immunofibroblast progenitors and induce the expansion of the fibroblast network, respectively. This supports the concept of fibroblast-targeting strategies to treat TLS-associated autoimmune diseases such as the SjS.

Conflict of interest

The author declares no conflict of interest.

Author details

Kerstin Klein[1,2]

1 Department of BioMedical Research, University of Bern, Bern, Switzerland

2 Department of Rheumatology and Immunology, University Hospital Bern, Bern, Switzerland

*Address all correspondence to: kerstin.klein@dbmr.unibe.ch; kerstin.klein@insel.ch

References

[1] Qin B, Wang J, Yang Z, Yang M, Ma N, Huang F, et al. Epidemiology of primary Sjogren's syndrome: a systematic review and meta-analysis. Ann Rheum Dis. 2015;74(11):1983-9.

[2] Mariette X, Criswell LA. Primary Sjogren's Syndrome. N Engl J Med. 2018;378(10):931-9.

[3] Shiboski CH, Shiboski SC, Seror R, Criswell LA, Labetoulle M, Lietman TM, et al. 2016 American College of Rheumatology/European League Against Rheumatism classification criteria for primary Sjogren's syndrome: A consensus and data-driven methodology involving three international patient cohorts. Ann Rheum Dis. 2017;76(1):9-16.

[4] Goules AV, Tzioufas AG. Primary Sjogren's syndrome: clinical phenotypes, outcome and the development of biomarkers. Immunol Res. 2017;65(1):331-44.

[5] Baer AN, Walitt B. Sjogren Syndrome and Other Causes of Sicca in Older Adults. Clin Geriatr Med. 2017;33(1):87-103.

[6] Manoussakis MN, Kapsogeorgou EK. The role of intrinsic epithelial activation in the pathogenesis of Sjogren's syndrome. J Autoimmun. 2010;35(3):219-24.

[7] Asam S, Neag G, Berardicurti O, Gardner D, Barone F. The role of stroma and epithelial cells in primary Sjogren's syndrome. Rheumatology (Oxford). 2019.

[8] Korsunsky I, Wei K, Pohin M, Kim EY, Barone F, Kang JB, et al. Cross-tissue, single-cell stromal atlas identifies shared pathological fibroblast phenotypes in four chronic inflammatory diseases. bioRxiv. 2021:2021.01.11.426253.

[9] Pitzalis C, Jones GW, Bombardieri M, Jones SA. Ectopic lymphoid-like structures in infection, cancer and autoimmunity. Nat Rev Immunol. 2014;14(7):447-62.

[10] Corsiero E, Nerviani A, Bombardieri M, Pitzalis C. Ectopic Lymphoid Structures: Powerhouse of Autoimmunity. Front Immunol. 2016;7:430.

[11] Jonsson MV, Skarstein K, Jonsson R, Brun JG. Serological implications of germinal center-like structures in primary Sjogren's syndrome. J Rheumatol. 2007;34(10):2044-9.

[12] Barone F, Bombardieri M, Manzo A, Blades MC, Morgan PR, Challacombe SJ, et al. Association of CXCL13 and CCL21 expression with the progressive organization of lymphoid-like structures in Sjogren's syndrome. Arthritis Rheum. 2005;52(6):1773-84.

[13] Lewis MJ, Barnes MR, Blighe K, Goldmann K, Rana S, Hackney JA, et al. Molecular Portraits of Early Rheumatoid Arthritis Identify Clinical and Treatment Response Phenotypes. Cell Rep. 2019;28(9):2455-70 e5.

[14] Antonioli L, Fornai M, Pellegrini C, Masi S, Puxeddu I, Blandizzi C. Ectopic Lymphoid Organs and Immune-Mediated Diseases: Molecular Basis for Pharmacological Approaches. Trends Mol Med. 2020;26(11):1021-33.

[15] Link A, Hardie DL, Favre S, Britschgi MR, Adams DH, Sixt M, et al. Association of T-zone reticular networks and conduits with ectopic lymphoid tissues in mice and humans. Am J Pathol. 2011;178(4):1662-75.

[16] Novkovic M, Onder L, Cupovic J, Abe J, Bomze D, Cremasco V, et al. Topological Small-World Organization of the Fibroblastic Reticular Cell

Network Determines Lymph Node Functionality. PLoS Biol. 2016;14(7):e1002515.

[17] Risselada AP, Kruize AA, Goldschmeding R, Lafeber FP, Bijlsma JW, van Roon JA. The prognostic value of routinely performed minor salivary gland assessments in primary Sjogren's syndrome. Ann Rheum Dis. 2014;73(8):1537-40.

[18] Risselada AP, Looije MF, Kruize AA, Bijlsma JW, van Roon JA. The role of ectopic germinal centers in the immunopathology of primary Sjogren's syndrome: a systematic review. Semin Arthritis Rheum. 2013;42(4):368-76.

[19] Theander E, Vasaitis L, Baecklund E, Nordmark G, Warfvinge G, Liedholm R, et al. Lymphoid organisation in labial salivary gland biopsies is a possible predictor for the development of malignant lymphoma in primary Sjogren's syndrome. Ann Rheum Dis. 2011;70(8):1363-8.

[20] Bombardieri M, Barone F, Lucchesi D, Nayar S, van den Berg WB, Proctor G, et al. Inducible tertiary lymphoid structures, autoimmunity, and exocrine dysfunction in a novel model of salivary gland inflammation in C57BL/6 mice. J Immunol. 2012;189(7):3767-76.

[21] Benezech C, White A, Mader E, Serre K, Parnell S, Pfeffer K, et al. Ontogeny of stromal organizer cells during lymph node development. J Immunol. 2010;184(8):4521-30.

[22] Cupedo T, Kraal G, Mebius RE. The role of $CD45^{+}CD4^{+}CD3^{-}$ cells in lymphoid organ development. Immunol Rev. 2002;189:41-50.

[23] Eberl G, Littman DR. The role of the nuclear hormone receptor RORgammat in the development of lymph nodes and Peyer's patches. Immunol Rev. 2003;195:81-90.

[24] Nayar S, Campos J, Smith CG, Iannizzotto V, Gardner DH, Mourcin F, et al. Immunofibroblasts are pivotal drivers of tertiary lymphoid structure formation and local pathology. Proc Natl Acad Sci U S A. 2019.

[25] Denton AE, Roberts EW, Linterman MA, Fearon DT. Fibroblastic reticular cells of the lymph node are required for retention of resting but not activated CD8+ T cells. Proc Natl Acad Sci U S A. 2014;111(33):12139-44.

[26] Novkovic M, Onder L, Bocharov G, Ludewig B. Graph Theory-Based Analysis of the Lymph Node Fibroblastic Reticular Cell Network. Methods Mol Biol. 2017;1591:43-57.

[27] Barone F, Nayar S, Campos J, Cloake T, Withers DR, Toellner KM, et al. IL-22 regulates lymphoid chemokine production and assembly of tertiary lymphoid organs. Proc Natl Acad Sci U S A. 2015;112(35):11024-9.

[28] Spadaro A, Rinaldi T, Riccieri V, Taccari E, Valesini G. Interleukin-13 in autoimmune rheumatic diseases: relationship with the autoantibody profile. Clin Exp Rheumatol. 2002;20(2):213-6.

[29] Mahlios J, Zhuang Y. Contribution of IL-13 to early exocrinopathy in $Id3^{-/-}$ mice. Mol Immunol. 2011;49(1-2):227-33.

[30] Belle I, Mahlios J, McKenzie A, Zhuang Y. Aberrant production of IL-13 by T cells promotes exocrinopathy in Id3 knockout mice. Cytokine. 2014;69(2):226-33.

[31] Lavoie TN, Stewart CM, Berg KM, Li Y, Nguyen CQ. Expression of interleukin-22 in Sjogren's syndrome: significant correlation with disease parameters. Scand J Immunol. 2011;74(4):377-82.

[32] Adams TS, Schupp JC, Poli S, Ayaub EA, Neumark N, Ahangari F,

et al. Single-cell RNA-seq reveals ectopic and aberrant lung-resident cell populations in idiopathic pulmonary fibrosis. Science advances. 2020;6(28):eaba1983.

[33] Habermann AC, Gutierrez AJ, Bui LT, Yahn SL, Winters NI, Calvi CL, et al. Single-cell RNA sequencing reveals profibrotic roles of distinct epithelial and mesenchymal lineages in pulmonary fibrosis. Science advances. 2020;6(28):eaba1972.

[34] Huang B, Chen Z, Geng L, Wang J, Liang H, Cao Y, et al. Mucosal Profiling of Pediatric-Onset Colitis and IBD Reveals Common Pathogenics and Therapeutic Pathways. Cell. 2019;179(5):1160-76 e24.

[35] Kinchen J, Chen HH, Parikh K, Antanaviciute A, Jagielowicz M, Fawkner-Corbett D, et al. Structural Remodeling of the Human Colonic Mesenchyme in Inflammatory Bowel Disease. Cell. 2018;175(2):372-86 e17.

[36] Martin JC, Chang C, Boschetti G, Ungaro R, Giri M, Grout JA, et al. Single-Cell Analysis of Crohn's Disease Lesions Identifies a Pathogenic Cellular Module Associated with Resistance to Anti-TNF Therapy. Cell. 2019;178(6):1493-508 e20.

[37] Mizoguchi F, Slowikowski K, Wei K, Marshall JL, Rao DA, Chang SK, et al. Functionally distinct disease-associated fibroblast subsets in rheumatoid arthritis. Nat Commun. 2018;9(1):789.

[38] Smillie CS, Biton M, Ordovas-Montanes J, Sullivan KM, Burgin G, Graham DB, et al. Intra- and Inter-cellular Rewiring of the Human Colon during Ulcerative Colitis. Cell. 2019;178(3):714-30 e22.

[39] Zhang F, Wei K, Slowikowski K, Fonseka CY, Rao DA, Kelly S, et al. Defining inflammatory cell states in rheumatoid arthritis joint synovial tissues by integrating single-cell transcriptomics and mass cytometry. Nat Immunol. 2019.

[40] Crowley T, Buckley CD, Clark AR. Stroma: the forgotten cells of innate immune memory. Clin Exp Immunol. 2018;193(1):24-36.

[41] Hall JC, Baer AN, Shah AA, Criswell LA, Shiboski CH, Rosen A, et al. Molecular Subsetting of Interferon Pathways in Sjogren's Syndrome. Arthritis & rheumatology. 2015;67(9):2437-46.

[42] Nezos A, Gravani F, Tassidou A, Kapsogeorgou EK, Voulgarelis M, Koutsilieris M, et al. Type I and II interferon signatures in Sjogren's syndrome pathogenesis: Contributions in distinct clinical phenotypes and Sjogren's related lymphomagenesis. J Autoimmun. 2015;63:47-58.

[43] Goldstein AS. A symbiotic relationship between epithelial and stromal stem cells. Proc Natl Acad Sci U S A. 2013;110(51):20356-7.

[44] Sequeira SJ, Larsen M, DeVine T. Extracellular matrix and growth factors in salivary gland development. Front Oral Biol. 2010;14:48-77.

[45] Bookman AA, Shen H, Cook RJ, Bailey D, McComb RJ, Rutka JA, et al. Whole stimulated salivary flow: correlation with the pathology of inflammation and damage in minor salivary gland biopsy specimens from patients with primary Sjogren's syndrome but not patients with sicca. Arthritis Rheum. 2011;63(7):2014-20.

[46] Leehan KM, Pezant NP, Rasmussen A, Grundahl K, Moore JS, Radfar L, et al. Minor salivary gland fibrosis in Sjogren's syndrome is elevated, associated with focus score and not solely a consequence of aging. Clin Exp Rheumatol. 2018;36 Suppl 112(3):80-8.

[47] Holmberg KV, Hoffman MP. Anatomy, biogenesis and regeneration of salivary glands. Monogr Oral Sci. 2014;24:1-13.

[48] Jonsson R, Kroneld U, Backman K, Magnusson B, Tarkowski A. Progression of sialadenitis in Sjogren's syndrome. Br J Rheumatol. 1993;32(7):578-81.

[49] Appel S, Le Hellard S, Bruland O, Brun JG, Omdal R, Kristjansdottir G, et al. Potential association of muscarinic receptor 3 gene variants with primary Sjogren's syndrome. Ann Rheum Dis. 2011;70(7):1327-9.

[50] Haldorsen K, Moen K, Jacobsen H, Jonsson R, Brun JG. Exocrine function in primary Sjogren syndrome: natural course and prognostic factors. Ann Rheum Dis. 2008;67(7):949-54.

[51] Pijpe J, Kalk WW, Bootsma H, Spijkervet FK, Kallenberg CG, Vissink A. Progression of salivary gland dysfunction in patients with Sjogren's syndrome. Ann Rheum Dis. 2007;66(1):107-12.

[52] Manoussakis MN, Spachidou MP, Maratheftis CI. Salivary epithelial cells from Sjogren's syndrome patients are highly sensitive to anoikis induced by TLR-3 ligation. J Autoimmun. 2010;35(3):212-8.

[53] Pringle S, Wang X, Verstappen G, Terpstra JH, Zhang CK, He A, et al. Salivary Gland Stem Cells Age Prematurely in Primary Sjogren's Syndrome. Arthritis & rheumatology. 2019;71(1):133-42.

[54] Kawakami M, Ishikawa H, Tachibana T, Tanaka A, Mataga I. Functional transplantation of salivary gland cells differentiated from mouse early ES cells in vitro. Hum Cell. 2013;26(2):80-90.

[55] Sfakis L, Kamaldinov T, Khmaladze A, Hosseini ZF, Nelson DA, Larsen M, et al. Mesenchymal Cells Affect Salivary Epithelial Cell Morphology on PGS/PLGA Core/Shell Nanofibers. Int J Mol Sci. 2018;19(4).

[56] Fauchais AL, Ouattara B, Gondran G, Lalloue F, Petit D, Ly K, et al. Articular manifestations in primary Sjogren's syndrome: clinical significance and prognosis of 188 patients. Rheumatology (Oxford). 2010;49(6):1164-72.

[57] Ramos-Casals M, Brito-Zeron P, Seror R, Bootsma H, Bowman SJ, Dorner T, et al. Characterization of systemic disease in primary Sjogren's syndrome: EULAR-SS Task Force recommendations for articular, cutaneous, pulmonary and renal involvements. Rheumatology (Oxford). 2015;54(12):2230-8.

[58] Lei L, Morgan S, Ntatsaki E, Ciurtin C. Comparative Assessment of Hand Joint Ultrasound Findings in Symptomatic Patients with Systemic Lupus Erythematosus and Sjogren's Syndrome: A Pilot Study. Ultrasound in medicine & biology. 2019;45(2):452-60.

[59] Ospelt C, Frank-Bertoncelj M. Why location matters – site-specific factors in rheumatic diseases. Nature reviews Rheumatology. 2017;13(7):433-42.

[60] Nygaard G, Firestein GS. Restoring synovial homeostasis in rheumatoid arthritis by targeting fibroblast-like synoviocytes. Nature reviews Rheumatology. 2020;16(6):316-33.